Praise for **In The Zone**

Being "in the zone" should be the rule, not the exception. A command performance — whether in the arts, athletics, or any other aspect of life — requires your total commitment. Ray Mulry's powerful and illuminating book, *In The Zone*, offers a specific methodology for reaching and maintaining your highest aspirations.

— *David N. Baker*
Distinguished Professor of Music, Indiana University
Joint Musical Director, Smithsonian Jazz Masterworks Orchestra

In The Zone hits on many fundamentals of sports with many concepts that should help any athlete — and should work equally well for "body" happiness in general. *In The Zone* teaches important concepts of stability, proper position and proper motion which any athlete needs; whether it is natural to them or needs to be relearned.

— *Walter Ray Williams, Jr.*
Professional Bowlers Association Hall of Fame
and Six Time Horseshoes World Champion

This is a fascinating "how to" book that can improve efficiency and increase pleasure in anyone's life. With simple, clear explanations of his basic principles, Ray Mulry triggers awareness that understanding and correct use of the body makes a vast difference in everything we do with both body and mind.

— *Sally Swift*
Internationally Recognized Equestrian Trainer
Author of The Centered Rider

In The Zone is the most cost-effective injury prevention program I have experienced. Viewing employees as "Industrial Athletes," Dr. Mulry's approach takes over where ergonomic improvements stop. It is a great guidebook for doing your best at whatever activity you choose.

— *Robert L. Beveridge*
Occupational Health & Safety Administrator, Northeast Utilities

World class athletes have always found their way into the "zone" of enhanced performance. Dr. Mulry's book unlocks and clearly explains these principles for everyone's benefit.

— *Rick Lee*
National Champion Boat Racer, Past World Record Holder

When you apply the basic building blocks of relaxation, balance, flexibility and focus, as presented in Dr. Mulry's book, and combine them with your own desire to succeed — you are well on your way to living your life In The Zone.

— *Chris Burford*
College Football Hall of Fame
Super Bowl Wide Receiver, Kansas City Chiefs Hall of Fame

All peak performers understand the importance of being in the zone. But Dr. Mulry does something totally new. He presents a clear and methodical way of how to get into that sweet spot. *In The Zone* is required reading for all of my martial arts trainers.

— *Sam Mason*
4th Degree Black Belt
National & International Martial Arts Champion

Dr. Mulry's *In The Zone* is a recipe for a happy, fulfilling life. He not only explains the importance of balancing our physical, mental and emotional being, he also shows us very specifically how, with simple exercises. Being "in the zone" is very important in all sports activities and in daily life. Dr. Mulry shows us how to get there in a way that everybody can understand and enjoy.

— *Helga Sable*
Gold Medalist, U.S. Women's Cross-Country Ski Team,
1995 World Masters Championship

In The Zone captures the essence of my profession, test flying and airshow performance. Relaxed, total focus is an absolute requirement if a pilot in my field is to survive. The need for these skills is multiplied and reinforced as the pilot progresses up the ladder to commercial, fighter pilot, or even astronaut. My compliments to Ray Mulry for stating the "secrets to success" in all walks of life.

— *G.P. Buzz Lynch*
Fellow in The Society of International Test Pilots

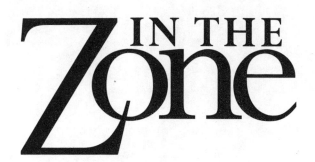

IN THE Zone

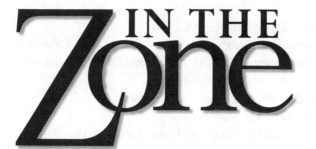

Making Winning Moments
Your Way of Life

Ray Mulry, Ph.D.

GREAT OCEAN PUBLISHERS
ARLINGTON, VIRGINIA

Book and cover design by M. M. Esterman
Illustrations by Margaret Park
Cover type and illustration by Bono Mitchell & Tom Specht

For information contact:

Great Ocean Publishers, Inc.
1823 North Lincoln Street
Arlington, Virginia 22207-3746

First Printing

Library of Congress Cataloging in Publication Data
Mulry, Ray.
    In the zone : making winning moments your way of life / Ray Mulry.
      p. cm.
    Includes bibliographical references.
    ISBN 0-915556-28-6 (pbk. : alk paper)
    1. Mind and body. 2. Mind and body -- Problems, exercises, etc.
3. Exercise -- Psychological aspects. 4. Self-actualization (Psychology)
5. New thought. I. Title.
BF161.M855   1995   95-34999
158'.1 --dc20

Contents

Illustrations

RELAXATION

BALANCE

FLEXIBILITY

FOCUS

LIVING IN THE ZONE

To

Βαρβαρα

of Athens

Acknowledgements

Authorship is ultimately a synergistic process, and I gratefully acknowledge the special people who have contributed to my life in such a manner:

My Irish father, poet of consummate style and wisdom ✧ My steadfast Norwegian mother, faithful to family, friends and self, enduring hardships, only she truly knows ✧ My daughter Kelly, and son, Marc — no father could be more proud ✧ Barbara, both balance and beam ✧ Mark and Margaret of Great Ocean Publishers, who provided support and clarity of vision.

IN THE ZONE

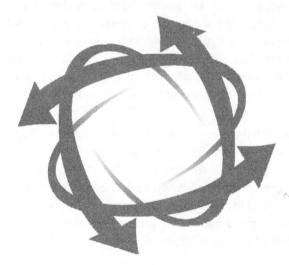

IN THE ZONE

What zone?

If you are at all involved with sports you may know what I mean right away. The zone is not a literal place — it's not the end zone on a football field. It's inside you, a feeling, a state of mind and body, a level of performance when everything clicks. You are effortlessly at your best.

Even if your athletic activities are limited to the couch and the TV set, you may know about being in the zone. It's the moment that often shows up on instant replays and sports highlights on the nightly news, the moment when the batter crushes a fastball with a towering home run to win the game in the bottom of the ninth, when a gymnast reaches down for that last ounce of strength and wins the gold on her final explosive vault.

Though the phrase comes from sports, the feeling of being in the zone is something we can all understand. In fact it has become a staple of TV commercials, where slow motion moments of high performance are used to sell everything from cars to beer and shoes to shampoo. Advertisers know that when we see someone performing at that level of excellence, we respond with admiration and excitement. We know we'd like to be there too.

Think of the times when you've had that feeling of total involvement — mental and physical — in what you were doing. Perhaps it's in the moment of driving a golf ball with coordination, ease and power, or dancing in complete harmony with the music and your partner, or giving a child a loving hug and kiss goodnight, or singing a hymn that expresses your deepest feelings of devotion. The possibilities are endless.

We've all had these exhilarating experiences. If you think about it, you might be able to remember such moments from your childhood, or recognize them in the lives of your own children. They may well be among the most memorable, the peak experiences of your life. So it's natural that we want to be in the zone — I'd say it's part of human nature.

Over the years, my work has brought me into contact with many high-performing individuals — athletes, executives, musicians, capable and talented persons in all walks of life — and many more who were not so fortunate or successful. I've observed them at work and play, and frequently tried to assist them, as a clinical psychologist in stress management and in developing wellness and fitness training programs.

No matter how vague their idea of being in the zone is, most of the people I meet and talk with understand two things about it. First, it occurs when we are totally involved, mentally and physically, in some activity we do well and enjoy. And second, it doesn't happen to most of us very often, and even when it does, it's unpredictable.

Eventually I came to the conclusion that common knowledge was accurate on the first point, and inaccurate on the second. The feeling of being in the zone occurs indeed when we are fully involved in what we are doing. But it need not be something that occurs by chance. In fact, there's a great deal we can do to make it happen.

After years of refining a comprehensive approach to correct body movement, I have concluded there are four crucial elements underlying high level performance: relaxation, balance, flexibility and focus.

You can easily see this pattern emerge in the observation of superior athletic performance. It simply cannot occur unless the body is relaxed, balanced, flexible and focused. When these factors are present, maximum energy efficiency is achieved, leaving more energy for greater strength and concentration. The energy of the total body system is not dissipated in tense muscles or mental distraction or fighting gravity. Rather, all available energy is devoted to performance of the task at hand.

It's partly a matter of biomechanics, as it is called by those who analyze the most minute physical details of top athletes' movements and muscles. Champions spend years of training developing certain muscles and refining body movements. Every move has to be characterized by power and efficiency of energy use.

Attaining physical mastery is more than a muscle development process. Advances in athletic training over the last several years show how great a part state of mind plays in athletic performance. Behind championship physical form is also a calm, centered, completely focused mind. There is a convergence of body and mind. You are relaxed balanced flexible and focused, working with maximum efficiency. If you're not at your best mentally, if you're nervous, uncentered, rigid or distracted, you simply cannot do your best.

Nervousness and distractibility are expensive. They shatter your attention and cost you energy. All brain processes and muscle movements are fueled by ATP (adenosine triphosphate), an energy releasing molecule that your body's cells make from the food you eat and the oxygen you breathe. Energy that could be available to better coordinate muscles, is often wasted on fruitless mental agitation.

When body and mind are working in relaxed, balanced, flexible and focused unison, you are approaching the peak of energy efficiency, and have prepared yourself to be — have put yourself into — the zone.

This applies to anything you might want to do in all the dimensions of your life, physically, socially, intellectually, professionally. The way we use our bodies can either assist self-mastery or prevent it. Through easily learned physical practices, you can achieve a calm and focused mental state. Through physical training you can bring your mind to a state of calm, centered and creative concentration that is crucial to mastery of any activity. This book will help you accomplish these goals.

In our culture we haven't fully appreciated the extent to

which mind and body influence one another. Other cultures are more mindful of this unity. Many oriental disciplines begin with the bodily basics, grounding the novice with correct breathing, posture, and movements. Whether it be in the martial arts or in painting, students spend much time learning good posture and paying attention to breathing and the quality of movements. Not until this foundation is in place do they advance to the particular techniques of their discipline.

In our society we tend to designate some experiences as mental and others as physical. We are now beginning to understand how mind and body are actually one. Many fields are beginning to apply this knowledge in ways that may be familiar to you. Mental preparation has become a vital part of athletic training. In medicine, much has been revealed about the powerful influence of the mind on physical health. Mental imagery has become a beneficial tool in the treatment of physical ailments. The military has determined that mental rehearsal of physical tasks nearly equals the learning value of actual exercise.

But can our bodies influence our minds? We may readily admit that our bodily feelings can influence our moods. Illness can create feelings of depression and poor self-esteem. But few of us fully appreciate the extent to which the body's experience actually shapes the mind from the very beginning of our lives. That is the picture that is gradually being clarified by research on the brain.

Our bodily experience plays a very large role in what we learn and how we think, because all of our learning is built upon the physical experience of our body. We come to know the world through our senses and our movements. How we think is shaped by what we have done.

When we are born, our brains are not complete. Only when the body begins to move and take in sensations do our brains really develop. The networks of nerve cells in our brains that allow us to think are created when nerve cells link together. They hook up with one another as we move, react, reflect. The dendrites of one cell grow to connect with other cells, creating extensive networks and routes. These networks grow in response to our physical movements.

That's how we first learn about gravity, for example. Repeated muscular movements become the base for more complex patterns of movement. Gradually we create the nerve system pathways for sitting, standing and walking. Our physical experience of gravity then lays the foundation for abstract thinking. The experience of falling, and of seeing other things fall, leads eventually to the very abstract notions of gravity — even to the understanding of planetary movements and beyond.

The complex, abstract ideas we can understand as adults are constructed on the building blocks of physical experience and understanding we gathered as children. As with gravity, the core concepts which are essential to the exhilarating experience of being in the zone — relaxation, balance, flexibility, and focus — are understandable and attractive to us because we learned and enjoyed them through our bodies as children, before we could name them.

So, in some ways the purpose of this book is to reintroduce you to what you already know. I am not referring to the wise rules and values we were all taught at home or in kindergarten, sturdy and deep though they may be. I mean those truths that are imbedded deep within us, but that we are not consciously aware of until something makes us think explicitly about them — truths we have learned through our bodies, our physical experience.

The effect of body on mind is not all in the distant past of childhood either. What your body does has a great role in shaping your mind and mood every single day. This is especially true when it comes to emotion, which is so completely felt and expressed by both mind and body. The very word emotion comes from the Latin roots *e*, meaning out and *movere*, to move. Whether you are happy or unhappy, your body language will reveal the truth.

Because our feelings are intrinsically body/mind experiences, emotional shifts can be brought about through either mental or physical intervention. A few years ago there was an interesting study done on smiling.[1] When research participants physically produced a smile, even a forced smile produced happier feelings; the physiological changes resulting from changes in facial muscles actually changed their mental state.

In the course of my work over the last few decades training thousands of people, I continually witness the power of the body to influence the mind. Following training in deep physical relaxation for example, I routinely observe greater openness of participants to learning. As their physical resistance and tensions are reduced, they become more emotionally receptive to change and often more mentally creative.

You can too. In writing this book, I wish to recreate the training so that you, in your own home and at your own pace, can learn the four basic elements of peak performance — and in the process learn how to get in the zone.

The book will take you through various body and mind exercises. First you will concentrate on learning with your body, the way you did as a child. Then out of the profound wisdom of the body will emerge a new understanding of what it means to be fully relaxed, balanced, flexible and focused. You will see ways to apply this knowledge in all sorts of activities, both at home and at work.

For this book to be effective, you must both read *and do the exercises*. They must be felt! Physical sensations are critically important to the learning process. Knowing what to do is not enough. You must read the exercises and then do them.

Try to keep in mind that in reading this book you are also studying yourself. This takes some time – time you are investing in your own self-development. The concepts and exercises may seem simple, and you may be tempted to glide past them. If you do, you will deprive yourself of opportunities to experience hidden benefits, benefits that can be gained only through actions, not words.

So get into some comfortable clothes and prepare yourself to move. Get back in touch with correct, energy efficient, strength maximizing, concentrated ways of moving. As you beome more relaxed, balanced, flexible and focused, you will be preparing your body and mind to be in the zone.

RELAXATION

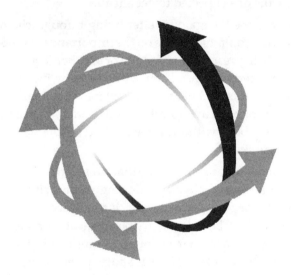

RELAXATION

A few decades ago, a visit to the doctor was often concluded with the generic advice, "You need to learn how to relax." That was good advice, except that few people knew how to do it, and many were not entirely sure they wanted to. There was a time, not so long ago, when the "high energy," tense, nervous personality was viewed as a productive, success-bound type. If you appeared somewhat frantic, short-tempered and busy doing something, you were the one expected to get ahead.

Then came the era of "better living through chemistry." Along with recommendations on the importance of relaxation, we were given prescriptions for one or another form of muscle relaxer or sleeping pill. Then with the growing interest in various meditation techniques, we explored "self-management" procedures for body and mind control. Today, you rarely pick up a self-help book without some method for the achievement of relaxation skills.

Most people are now aware that a relaxed mind and body are essential for effective functioning in any situation, and particularly for peak performance. It might seem paradoxical that we need to be relaxed to perform at our best under pressure, but it's a truth we're often reminded of. Think of all the slow motion replays of great sports performances you've seen on TV. Even if you're not a sports fan, you've probably seen those highlighted moments so frequently replayed on the news: amazing diving catches, crushing swings of baseball bat and golf club, basketball players levitating above the rim with seemingly timeless grace, gymnasts perfectly at ease on the very edge of danger and disaster.

Top athletes are often very articulate and eloquent about how relaxed they feel at these moments when they are in the zone of peak performance. Their feelings and state of mind mirror their physical ease, and are actually inseparable from their physical skills. And, though few of us use our bodies in such conscious and visible ways, sports and physical activity are an excellent way into understanding and experiencing the four elements which are key to being in the zone in any activity in our lives: relaxation, balance, flexibility and focus.

Keep in mind that when I use the term relaxation in this book, I am not referring to a sleepy, or fuzzy state of consciousness. I am referring to alert relaxation -- the state of mind variously described as inner stillness, clarity of consciousness, sense of readiness, keenness of perception. It is when we function without interference from within or without, ready and prepared to focus. Our senses are alive and we are prepared for effective action. We are calm, yet fully able to deal with ongoing circumstances. We are separate, yet in touch with things around us; we cooperate rather than resist; move forward, rather than backward; look for the positive, gliding past the negative; think of possibilities rather than obstacles. We are open to multiple alternatives. We feel hopeful, and experience a general sense of well being.

Does this sound like the way you feel right now, or most of the time, or any time you want to? Probably not, if you're like most of us. But that doesn't mean you can't.

RELAXED BODY

The easiest path to a relaxed state of mind is through a relaxed body. So here's something to try right now. As you do the following exercise, keep in mind that you cannot be relaxed and tense at the same time. Relaxation and tension are mutually incompatible states; one survives at the expense of the other. Try it to see if it works for you.

RELAXATION VS. TENSION

Clench both of your fists to the count of ten.

Relax your fist and notice the difference. You can feel the muscles as they relax and you can even feel the blood returning. Your palms might even feel warm.

Now, place your elbows out in front of you and press your palms against each other. Push hard and continue to the count of ten. Release and notice how the muscles relax in your hands, arms and shoulders.

The exercise you have just tried is an illustration of a basic principle of many muscle relaxation training programs. If you did this tension versus relaxation procedure with each of your muscles, one at a time, you would become more aware of tension in specific parts of your body and how to reduce it.

Now that medical experts have confirmed the harmful, even dangerous effects of stress, we are more alert to its pervasive presence in our lives. A decade ago, I would ask seminar participants whether physical tension was a concern of theirs. Most were reluctant to admit to this, even though they probably felt tension in their personal and/or professional lives. It was as though they were admitting to personal weakness. When I ask this same question today, participants readily discuss their tensions.

Even though we are now more willing to admit to tension in our lives, many of us don't fully grasp how tense we often are. We have the "idea" that we are tense but don't "feel" these tensions directly. We accept tension as a routine part of our lives, and this wears us down over time. It is an inefficiency factor in our functioning. Tense, tight muscles work less effectively and require greater effort, causing us to feel needlessly tired at the end of the day.

We express our tensions in our appearance as well as in our behaviors. When tense, we are inclined toward short temper, irritability, snap judgments, needless arguments, and our interpersonal lives are fraught with conflict. We feel physically uncomfortable, and are also more prone to illness and injuries of all sorts. So, a big first step toward relaxation is to recognize and eliminate the tension in your own body. Coordination of breathing with conscious relaxation of muscles helps you to achieve this.

BREATHING

Whatever activity your mind and body may be engaged in, there is one thing you are certainly doing at this very moment: breathing. From our first breath at birth, to our final exhalation at the end of life, nothing is more basic to the life process than this breathing which brings life-giving oxygen to our bodies.

Fortunately for us, normal breathing does not require effort or self-discipline. Our autonomic nervous system allows us to continue our breathing without conscious effort. But how about consciously using our breathing for enhanced relaxation, tension management and even peak performance?

Athletes and other people who perform under pressure frequently mention the power of breathing to aid us in getting into the zone of high performance. Describing the "natural athlete" in all of us, world champion gymnast and university coach Dan Millman writes in *The Inner Athlete*,[1]

> The breath is a key to your emotional state, because it both reflects — and can control — your level of tension. Learning to breathe properly, with full feeling, gives you the ability quite literally to "inspire" yourself. The natural athlete, like the infant, breathes naturally, from deep in the body, with slow, full, relaxed, and balanced inhalations and exhalations.

What is true for top performing athletes is true for you. This is a theme we shall return to frequently. But, in keeping with our principle that experience is the key to real understanding, let's begin by practicing a skill that will serve as a foundation for many of the abilities you will master through this book.

SOFT STOMACH BREATHING

To explore your breathing, sit with a straight, vertical back (as opposed to a slumping position). Take a deep breath as you inhale through your nose. Hold it.

Did you pull your stomach in, or did you push it out? *Now exhale.* A common response is, "I pulled my stomach in." This is not what you want to do. When you pull your stomach in, you restrict space needed by your lungs for full expansion. So, try another breath, only this time, "push your stomach out" as you gradually inhale:

Slowly inhale through your nose to the count of four, pushing your stomach out. Hold it briefly. Slowly exhale through your mouth to the count of eight, and relax.

This is actually the way you breathe as you sleep. It is natural for your stomach to slowly expand and then relax into a flat stomach position. We call this **Soft Stomach Breathing**.

Do three more deep Soft Stomach Breaths. Notice the feeling of relaxation gradually settling over you. Your heart rate is slowing down. Your blood pressure is decreasing. You feel less pressured. You are reducing physical tension. Soft Stomach Breathing is easy to do and can be done anytime during your day. Take a few Soft Stomach Breaths now and then, especially when you feel pressured and tense. When you practice this behavior over time, you will develop a life-giving habit.

THE POSITION OF COMFORT

To further develop your relaxation skills through deep breathing, you want a suitable resting position. Since lying down reduces downward pull of gravity on your body, take advantage of this by using deep breathing in the **Position of Comfort**.[2] The position is as follows:

Lie on your back and place a pillow or two under your knees. This flattens your lower back. A small pillow or a rolled towel under your neck will also give you valuable support. This will help you relax with your spine in a straight line position. Rest your hands lightly on your stomach or by your side, whichever is most comfortable.

If you are uncomfortable lying on your back, which can happen if you have low back pain resulting from a bulging spinal disc, you can still use the Position of Comfort. Just turn onto your side and be sure your spine is straight and your knees bent. If your waist is narrower than your hips and shoulders, causing you to sag at the waist, a straight spine can be achieved by placing a pillow at the waistline for support.

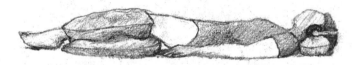

The Position of Comfort with Pillows

A word of caution for those with rheumatoid arthritis in the knees. People with rheumatoid arthritis, who spend prolonged periods of time in the bent knee position, can develop contractures. Contractures occur when knee joints tighten and you have trouble straightening your legs. If you have this condition, you can still use the bent knee position during relaxation exercises which typically last only about a half hour or so.

Also, a word of caution for pregnant women. After the fifth month of gestation, lying on your back for too long can put pressure from the uterus on to the major blood vessels, compromising circulation to the baby. To avoid this, try lying on your side.

In summary, The Position of Comfort is a horizontal

resting position, providing relief from the downward pull of gravity on your spine. It is useful for most people and requires your back be straight, and your knees bent. Deep Soft Stomach Breathing in this position is very relaxing.

TAKE SOME TIME OUT RIGHT NOW

It will be useful to take some time out from reading to experience how it feels to deeply relax. Those so inclined can do the following:

Lie down in the Position of Comfort. Support your legs with pillows. Support your neck with a rolled up towel or something similar. Do several Soft Stomach Breaths.

Allow yourself to gradually enter a deep state of relaxation.

THE EFFECTS OF RELAXATION

If you have experienced Soft Stomach Breathing in the Position of Comfort as suggested, you will have experienced the benefits of relaxation in a way that is more real than words and scientific knowledge can make it. But a scientific understanding of the effects of relaxation on our bodies makes it easier to see why relaxation is so beneficial.

When you deeply relax, several important physiological events occur in your body. Among these healthful changes are:

> Heart rate slows down
>
> Blood pressure lowers
>
> Muscles relax
>
> Blood vessels dilate
>
> Blood passes more freely throughout your body
>
> Oxygen consumption is enhanced
>
> Waste products are eliminated with greater efficiency
>
> Your body's natural production of healthful chemicals increases

Stress reduction is a much publicized health care goal.

Word of the beneficial effects has started to spread. But the far-reaching benefits are even more extensive than is commonly known. For example, when you consider that the brain accounts for only one fiftieth of the body's weight but uses one fifth of the body's oxygen supply, you can see how increased blood circulation makes for more efficient thought processing.[3]

Similarly, when the body is under stress, it produces a variety of chemicals to protect itself. These chemicals, notably adrenalin, perform very crucial functions such as tensing our muscles for fight or flight, and increasing our sensitivity to any external stimuli which might signal danger. But continued stress, with continued high levels of adrenalin, can have harmful effects on both body and mind. It increases our vulnerability to illness and infection, lowers our threshold of irritability and aggressive behavior, and decreases our ability to think clearly, learn and remember. It is a major contributor to the growing list of symptoms which are labeled "learning disorders." Adrenalin is a response to life-threatening situations, not meant to be a sustained influence on our actions and state of mind.

Interestingly, our bodies secrete other life-preserving chemicals when we are under stress. For example interferons and interleukins which raise cell polarity and enhance their resistance to disease, are the body's health-giving and longevity-inducing response to stress. According to endocrinologist, Deepak Chopra, and other writers on the subject of stress, our emotions can influence and reduce the harmful effects of stress.[4] When we accept stressful situations as positive challenges, adventures, or opportunities for growth, and take positive steps to manage the stress, we promote the production of the more beneficial brain and body chemistry.[5] The recent and continuing discovery of such substances in the brain, confirms what many people have believed about the delicate interplay between mind, emotions and body. It also makes it clear that what seem like small adjustments of both physical and mental habits can have profound effects.

USING RELAXATION TO GET IN THE ZONE

I once asked a world-renowned martial artist how he uses his breathing during competition. "When I enter the ring," he answered, "I take a deep breath to relax and center myself. Then I focus on my opponent and look for signs of tension. His tensions reveal his weaknesses." This highly trained athlete competes in the most difficult competition in the martial arts, bare knuckle fighting with no rules. There is no luck; nothing but concentration, and skill. In these challenging circumstances, he takes a deep breath before he does anything else. By being relaxed and centered, he is better prepared to meet the challenges before him.

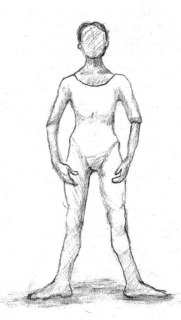

"Relaxation Equals the Peak of Efficiency"

Ballet may seem worlds away from bare knuckle fighting, but it's fascinating to see how the same emphasis on breathing and relaxation are essential to both. All good dance instructors, for example, teach proper breathing and relaxation. Dancers must be able to breathe uninterruptedly, evenly and deeply, allowing for greatest intake of oxygen. As Nikolai Tarasov writes, in *Ballet Technique For The Male Dancer*,[6]

> It is necessary always to make sure that the pupils inhale and exhale — despite any acceleration — as uninterruptedly, deeply, and evenly as possible, and that they not become unnecessarily upset or tighten the muscles — especially those of the face, neck and shoulders.

Dancers, who are aware of the subtle interplay of grace and strength, know that muscle tension affects not only the visual effect of the dancer's performance, but the dancer's physical efficiency. "Relaxation equals the peak of efficiency," is the way Leonard Fowler of The Fowler School of Classical Ballet put it. To make the same point, track coach D. Bruce Lockerbie states: "The essence of success in running lies in obtaining a maximum of strength from a minimum of effort. To achieve this equation, a coach urges relaxation in the running form."[7]

Experienced, knowledgeable athletes can often tell at a glance whether a fellow athlete is performing at peak efficiency. When the most recent Olympics were televised, expert commentators were instantly predicting how well star runners would do even in the shortest dashes simply by observing how relaxed their bodies were as they ran. Physical relaxation opens pathways within the body. As we allow blood to flow more freely through our arteries and capillaries, it carries oxygen more effectively into muscle tissue. Oxygen is the life force of muscle tissue, just as it is the life force of all living things.

Relaxation is just as important to the finest, most precise muscular activities under extreme pressure as it is in the flat-out total effort of the 100 meter dash in the Olympic finals. Here's what an expert has to say about precise muscular activities during the moment of pulling the trigger in rifle marksmanship:

> The ability of a marksman to keep a rifle steady

during the short space of time that the action in the breech mechanism takes place is known as "holding." ... Good "holding" can be attributed to good breathing. It is necessary in all shooting positions to breathe slowly and deeply. Make every effort to subdue internal excitement, if it is present. Such excitement or nervousness naturally causes the heart to beat faster, making breathing abnormal and the pulse beat more rapid, all of which affects your holding and aim.[8]

You don't have to be interested in shooting or in marksmanship to see how your breathing could effect your coordination and your aim. You don't even have to get out of your chair. Try this:

Imagine you have a rifle in your hands. Choose a target—a door knob across the room, for example, or an object outside the window. Slowly inhale as you raise the rife to your shoulder to aim. Bring your sights in alignment with the target, then slowly exhale until your lungs are nearly empty. When you have a clear picture of the target, again slowly inhale with a Soft Stomach Breath until your lungs are about half full and hold the breath momentarily as you slowly squeeze the trigger. Immediately after making the shot, continue slow, deep breathing.

People are not the only sensitive observers of tension in their fellow humans. As many pet owners can testify, animals are extremely aware of our body language — it's really the language we share with them. So horseback riding provides an intriguing insight into the linkage of breathing, relaxation and performance. In her book *Centered Riding,*[9] Sally Swift maintains that the horse is sensitive to tensions and imbalances of the rider and responds to them with resistance. To overcome this problem, she teaches correct breathing as one of Four Basics of correct riding technique.

You can breathe a horse to quietness. You can breathe him past things that scare him. If you hold your breath as you come to that big rock, he'd say, "She's frightened! There must be gremlins there." But if you keep breathing or talking (you can't hold your breath when you are talking), it gives him confidence. Breathing must be done without tension. Allow it to be constant and rhythmical. Holding your breath blocks the suppleness in certain parts of your body. And remember to breathe though your whole body.

BUT WHAT IF YOU DON'T RIDE HORSES?

Are you convinced that "Relaxation equals the peak of efficiency"? I find that most people are willing to accept this proposition in theory, but in fact it runs counter to the way they act day to day, not to mention in pressure situations. The idea that we rise to a challenge by tensing up and holding our breath is deeply ingrained in our habitual ways of thinking. It is deeply embedded in our body's learned habits as well.

If you want to feel the difference between moving while tense versus moving with relaxed muscles and continuous breathing, try this exercise:

Go onto your knees and prepare to do a push-up on the floor. Put your hands on the floor and then straighten your back and legs. You are now in the push-up position. Now tense all your muscles, hold your breath and do two push-ups.

Now return to your knees and take a short rest. Do a few soft stomach breaths.

You are now rested and relaxed. Try the push-ups again. Stay fully relaxed and inhale as your body descends to the floor. Exhale slowly as you push up with your arms. Do two of these.

You are now more aware of how physical tension and holding your breath while exerting yourself is both tiring and ineffective. One or two push-ups, done in a tense manner, can cause you to feel flushed and even light headed.

So perhaps I should ask: even though you find these examples convincing, do you really believe they apply to you? Perhaps you don't ride horses, or do ballet? You avoid running, even for a bus, and your bare knuckle fighting days are far behind you? Is there some way you can **experience** the actuality of these notions so that you can get the benefit of them?

Try this simple experiment with a friend:

Stand up. Extend one of your arms straight out from your shoulder, perpendicular to your body. Make your arm as tense as you can, from the muscles of the shoulder, through your forearm, all the way down to your clenched fist.

Now ask your friend to try to force your arm back down to your side as you resist.

Rest a moment. Now repeat the challenge, with this variation: Instead of tensing up as you resist, relax. Do not stop your breathing; rather, let it continue as Soft Stomach Breathing. And instead of tightening the muscles in your shoulder, arm and hand, relax them. As you hold your arm straight out, imagine it has a steel bar running through its entire length (you might want to picture that in your mind) — imagine that it is a steel bar. Keep your muscles relaxed and continue your Soft Stomach Breathing.

Now ask your friend to try again to force your arm back down to your side.

What difference did you find in the two different tests? *Don't* read on yet. Try exchanging places with your friend. Are the results the same?

I don't want to influence the outcome of this experiment, or deprive you of the chance of discovering it for yourself, but I'm sure it won't surprise you that I expect you will find the second method of counteracting the force on your arm was more successful. That is in fact what most people do experience. But people are frequently surprised at this result, even — or especially—when they experience it through their own bodies.

We can believe, in theory, that a relaxed body and a strong mental attitude are more powerful than merely tensed muscles. But without experiencing the theory in action, it's hard to really connect with it ourselves, or to know how to put it into action in our own lives.

CHANGE YOUR BODY TO CHANGE YOUR MIND

The fact that our minds and bodies are deeply interconnected is something we know intuitively. Medical and neuroscientific research is deepening that understanding with new discoveries at an ever-increasing rate. Yet too few of us use this knowledge in ways that can improve our lives.

In the case of relaxation, we can use our knowledge of techniques like Soft Stomach Breathing to change our physical state. It's also important to see that **by changing our physical state, we are changing our mental state as well.** It's a two way street. Body expresses and influences mind. Mind directs but also responds to changes in the physical state.

We can witness these powerful cross influences directly. For example, it doesn't take long to figure out that a person is mentally agitated or fearful. You can sense it instantly through physical signs. Jumpiness, quavering of the voice, distractibility, inability to hold eye contact — in extremes, elevated heart rate, sweating and fast breathing — these are the symptoms of a body and mind on red alert.

You would need these heightened sensitivities and capacities to survive in a tiger infested forest, but in the usual course of life, they get in the way and project something other than self-confidence.

You can bring these physical manifestations under control through Soft Stomach Breathing and relaxation. As we've already seen, deep breathing lowers blood pressure and slows heart rate. The relaxing nervous system stops sending distress messages to the muscles and sense organs. Feelings of agitation or nervousness are replaced with a quiet calm. Body and mind together recover equanimity and project physical and mental steadiness.

Soft Stomach Breathing can be a powerful tool in all situations. Relax through deep breathing whenever you feel yourself becoming agitated, nervous or overwrought. If you feel frustration mounting or anger rising, stop and take Soft Stomach Breaths until you are calm again. Whenever you are nervous and want to bolster self-confidence take a few deep Soft Stomach Breaths and prepare yourself for a good performance.

USES IN DAILY LIFE

Most of us never have to fight tigers, few people face real danger on a daily basis. Yet all of us encounter fear about one thing or another. There is one quite common situation in daily life which seems to many of us to be the civilized equivalent of fighting tigers. It might surprise you — or, then again, it might not — that according to opinion polls our number one cultural phobia is public speaking.

PUBLIC SPEAKING

In front of an audience, you want your message to be convincing and enjoyable. Relaxed speakers connect with the audience. Tense speakers "sound" out of control, just as they "look" out of control. We speak with our voice, and we speak with our body. Lack of voice control, jerky movements, restlessness and so on are observable behaviors that make audiences uneasy. Nervous behavior distracts from the presentation because the audience focuses on the speaker's emotions.

Contrast this with the relaxed, flowing, coordinated, body language of self-confident speakers, fully in command of self and audience. Verbal and physical presentations are coordinated, leading the audience's attention to the central message. Audiences can be captivated by the concert of coordinated actions and words. The performance is pleasing to the eye and to the ear. As with a gymnast or a dancer, a relaxed, powerful performance is possible when you take advantage of correct breathing techniques.

IMAGINE THIS

You are about to give a speech. You are waiting to be introduced to the audience. You hear your name mentioned along with various accomplishments. You feel uneasiness in your stomach and are short of breath. You feel tension in your neck and shoulders and feel pressured. Your heart rate is increasing, your hands are trembling, and the more you feel yourself losing control, the worse things get.

You need control over the situation. Take a deep Soft Stomach Breath, slowly exhale and relax. Take two more breaths and notice how nervousness changes to relaxed centeredness. Remember, "It is impossible to be relaxed and tense at the same time."

RELAXING YOUR VOICE

The stress of public speaking can greatly impact your breathing and vocal production. A common reaction to panic is difficulty breathing. When this happens, breathing is fast and shallow, reducing air flow in and out of the lungs. Chest muscles tighten and the diaphragm can't function as it should.

Public speaking may not quite send you into a panic attack, but if you are unable to relax, your voice will expose your nervousness. Soft Stomach Breathing facilitates a relaxed, focused and effective speaking style. Understanding how correct breathing affects voice quality and projection will improve your presentations.

Experts on vocalization consider correct breathing and a relaxed body vital to use of the voice in both singing and speaking.[10] When you take a deep breath, the diaphragm (one of the largest muscles in the body located between the chest and the abdominal cavity) is called into action. As you inhale, this muscle is pulled down, pushing the walls of your abdominal cavity outward. Naturally, any tendency to tighten abdominal muscles, restricts your ability to take a deep breath. As the diaphragm drops down during Soft Stomach Breathing, spreading of the rib cage and back also occurs. This overall process creates a vacuum in your lungs, drawing air inward. Once you have inhaled in this manner, you can then exhale. As you exhale, your diaphragm relaxes and returns to the original position.

Think of your diaphragm as a bellows that opens and pulls air in, then closes pushing air out. Your voice is like a musical instrument. It needs adequate air flow to produce quality sound, so breath control is essential.

NOW, TRY GIVING A SPEECH

Imagine you are about to give a speech.

First, take a deep breath, so you have a chest full of air and then say, "Welcome Everyone!"

Second, exhale most of the air from your lungs and then say, "Welcome Everyone!"

In the first situation you feel in control. In the second situation, your voice is weak. The reason is explained by another expert in voice production:

> The actual production of tone should follow — grow out of — breath control, and not precede it. That is, the conditions which should prevail during the act of singing are dependent almost entirely upon breath action, and can best be established through a careful study of breathing before the act of singing is undertaken.... Failure to properly control breath before and during the act of singing causes pressure at the larynx, giving rise to stiffness of jaw and tongue and lack of control over the tone.[11]

Correct breathing during singing or speaking should never involve straining throat or vocal organs. Soft Stomach Breathing and relaxation are essential to voice control and excellence of tone. If you want to improve your voice quality, develop correct breathing habits.

If you want to learn how to breathe more effectively, try the following:

IMPROVE YOUR BREATHING

To gain better control of your diaphragm - exhale (push) all of the air from your lungs. Exhale until your stomach muscles are hard. Don't inhale until you have to. Now let go of your stomach muscles and let the air come rushing in automatically. Do this a few more times and then relax for a moment.

The next exercise will give you a better sense of rhythm during breathing.

As you walk across the room, inhale with a Soft Stomach Breath during your first four steps, hold your breath for the next four steps, then fully exhale during the next six steps; walk four more steps before starting over again — inhale, hold, exhale, hold.

To learn more about your breathing and how it can be coordinated with full body movements, simply change your breathing by walking faster or slower.

LONG INHALES AND LONG EXHALES

You can increase your total volume of intake by practicing long inhales. In so doing, you will be using more of your lungs. To achieve this, slowly inhale as you take a deep Soft Stomach Breath. Hold it for a short period of time and slowly exhale.

BREATH CONTROL

A flexible and well controlled diaphragm is essential for increased breath control. This exercise will help you develop breath control by "panting."

Raise your elbows up high to the top of your head, lifting your shoulders and your chest. (This locks your chest and forces you to use your diaphragm). Relax your hands behind your neck, open your mouth and stick your tongue out as far as you can. Take a deep soft stomach breath and then exhale ... start slowly and gradually breathe faster. Soon you will be taking quick, short breaths and this is called panting.

Practicing the fundamentals of correct breathing makes a

difference. Recently, our training organization conducted a program for a group of employees of a utility company. A few days later, I asked one of the participants whether he had used any of the recommended techniques. He certainly had, he said enthusiastically: he had introduced Soft Stomach Breathing to his Barbershop Quartet. They practiced breathing exercises for forty-five minutes prior to singing. Afterwards they were able to sustain notes with higher levels of voice control than ever before.

Soft Stomach Breathing, also called diaphragmatic breathing, is taught in many walks of life. Women learn diaphragmatic breathing in preparation for childbirth, Yoga practitioners to relax during stretching, Tai Chi students for centeredness and overall effectiveness, and the list goes on. Many competitive athletes engage in some form of relaxed breathing exercises as a part of their overall training.

The simple fact is, relaxed, centered people perform more effectively than people who are tense, tight and restricted. To quote the great teacher of acting, Constantin Stanislavsky, "The rhythm, which every man has to express in life, originates from his breathing and, consequently, from his entire organism, from his first need, without which life is impossible."

INSOMNIA

Millions of people have difficulty going to sleep at night. The scenario goes something like this: "I feel tense and restless. I am thinking about activities of the day, unresolved problems, things to be done. My mind is racing. I want to go to sleep, but I can't. I try my repertoire of tricks for falling asleep, but they are not working. What are my options?"

One option is to take a sleeping pill, but this tends to be counterproductive in the long run. Sleeping pills, like alcohol, interfere with good, natural sleep. They tend to suppress REM time, the valuable time during sleep when the brain consumes large quantities of vital oxygen. What can you do to relax?

Try lying on your back in the Position of Comfort, with a pillow or two under your knees. Support the curve in your neck with a small pillow or rolled up towel. You have elevated and supported your knees, which flattens and relaxes your neck, shoulders and back. Concentrate on Soft Stomach Breathing as you relax into the Position of Comfort. Continue to do this and you will gradually fall asleep.

Don't be concerned if you don't fall asleep as rapidly as you would like. You'll soon discover that the more you practice, the more reliably Soft Stomach Breathing will produce a state of relaxation. Don't feel you must remain in the Position of Comfort all night long. We naturally change our sleeping position forty to sixty times throughout the night.

SELF-CONFIDENCE

Correct breathing and relaxation are unquestionably crucial to effectiveness in a wide range of activities, and consequently to our overall sense of ourselves. Our sense of personal effectiveness and self-worth is directly related to what we do and how well we do it. So when we ask, "Who am I?" we are also asking, "What do I do well?" Every skill, every discipline requires study and practice, some fields requiring years to master. Performance at any step along the way will be improved by relaxation skills.

As we can clearly see in activities like ballet and athletics, inner calmness and self-confidence increase as level of skill increases. Self-confidence comes from experience. As the quiet mind and relaxed muscles of self-confident performers react with swifter reflex, so do tensions of the less skilled further prepare for defeat. Relaxation helps but you just can't fake self-confidence. If you are unskilled, unprepared, self-doubting, afraid and restricted, you'd best take a good look at yourself and make needed changes.

DEVELOPING A RELAXED STANCE TOWARD OTHERS

Self-acceptance occurs when you say to yourself, "I like

who I am and what I am becoming." You like yourself when you follow your interests and develop your talents. As you become more relaxed and self-confident, you become more accepting of other people and other living things. Because life is a growing process, self-acceptance and acceptance of others is a developing process. Kindness, recognition of the needs of others, acceptance of other living things, develop gradually along with your gradually maturing self. When you treat other living things with the same consideration you give yourself, you are well on your way toward a relaxed, accepting way of living.

When you "breathe deeply" you open yourself to new sources of influence. The most obvious of these, is life-giving oxygen. The more you are open to new experiences and allow yourself to absorb and learn, the more you grow. A relaxed, open attitude leads to greater exposure to evolving life experiences because you are receptive to new ideas and new ways of doing things.

There is an ongoing process in nature: living things are typically growing, or they are dying. Relaxed, open, people enjoy growth and change. They plant and water seeds and trust nature to complete the process. When you are relaxed and trusting of yourself, you tend also to trust others. Your trusting attitude creates an atmosphere conducive to growth for everyone involved. This is as true in the home as in the workplace.

COUNTERACTING STRESS

In stressful environments, the relaxed openness you wish to cultivate may seem impossible to maintain. Tension generally breeds further tension. Nothing spreads faster than frazzled nerves and short tempers. Today the typically overcommitted, overworked lifestyle ratchets up the stress levels in the environment. Everyone can benefit by cultivating relaxation skills and seeking soothing environments.

A change of environment can spark much needed personal

refueling. Albert Einstein, for example, sought environments both relaxing and inspiring. He enjoyed escape into music and there was always his interest in sailing and the lightness of spirit resulting from the wind and water. He always took a notebook with him. When the wind would settle, he would turn to his thoughts. With relaxation would often come the solution to a perplexing problem. Einstein's preoccupation with sailing came from his fascination with the counterplay of wind and water. He had no interest in motor driven boats, and no interest in competition. It was the naturalness, the relaxation, the flow of nature, that led him always to return to sailing and the sea as a source of joy and creativity.

Henri Poincaré, the gifted French mathematician and scientist, frustrated with his lack of success in his path toward discovery of Fuchsian functions, left the city for the seaside to relax and think of other things. While walking the shore, an idea surfaced with unexpected suddenness and clarity. It proved to be the key to his great mathematical discovery. Poincaré ascribes this inspirational process to the working of his unconscious during periods of rest following periods of intense work.

If highly disciplined individuals like Einstein and Poincaré require a restful, soothing environment to bring out their best thoughts, then surely the rest of us can benefit from such settings too. In fact most of us seek a variety of pleasant environments and influences and there can be little doubt they can and do stir our creative spirits.

RELAXATION AND AUDITORY PERCEPTION

Environmental sounds have a great effect on our ability to relax. Soft sounds, sounds with rhythms slow and peaceful, have different effects than do harsh sounds with uncoordinated rhythms, clashing tones and the like. All too familiar are ringing telephones, barking dogs, screeching tires, honking horns, loud music, and the list goes on. Consider your home, a retreat meant to be comfortable and relaxed, and then consider how much attention you pay to sounds throughout your home and how they affect you.

People hear better when they are relaxed and this leads to new sensations and information. Try this exercise:

Select a specific sound within your immediate environment. Focus on it and become fully aware of its qualities. It has pitch, rhythm, speed, intensity. As you intensify your focus, you will gradually drown out other sounds. When concentration is fully focused on that one, specific sound, you will not notice other sounds.

Take some Soft Stomach Breaths and gradually relax. Continue your attention to the sound you selected, but allow other sounds to enter your space. Allow yourself to alternate attention from the focal sound to other sounds, never completely abandoning attention to the focal sound.

This experience is similar to listening to a symphony. You may have a favorite instrument you like to focus on, yet want also to hear the complete symphony. You want the specific and you want the general. When you are relaxed and use your senses in this manner, your theater of experience is richer, more rewarding and informative.

RELAXATION AND VISUAL PERCEPTION

Martial artists train themselves to be aware of what they call "hard eyes" and "soft eyes." With hard eyes, your visual focus narrows and your concentration is intensely focused on a specific thing. This is very useful at times. With soft eyes, your focus is wide, your peripheral vision is enlarged. Soft eyes lead to a wider net of information and a wider platform for action. When your outlook is relaxed and your focus wide, you can gather more information from the world around you.

Select an object in your immediate environment to focus on. Study it carefully and examine the elements that make it what it is. Notice the shape, color, and anything else that comes to your attention. Focused attention leads to enhanced awareness of detail and structure.

Now, take a few Soft Stomach Breaths and allow your perception to broaden as you relax. Continue your attention to the object, but allow yourself to perceive other things within your 180 degree perceptual span. This requires a relaxed, open attitude, both in body and mind.

A QUIET PLACE AND SOLITUDE

Your personal space is an undefined area surrounding you, bordered by invisible boundaries; it is the amount of space you need to avoid feeling crowded and invaded. The amount of personal space you need and the time you need in that space, varies from day to day as your tensions rise and fall. Adequate personal space is a psychological requirement and without it, you can become increasingly irritable and uncentered.

Recognizing your need for a quiet place is important; the place itself could be a den, workshop, garden, bedroom, or anywhere a feeling of pleasant solitude is available on a predictable basis. Your retreat gives you important time with yourself. This is not an anti-social gesture, but a chance to collect yourself. As Henry David Thoreau wrote in **Walden,** "I have a great deal of company in my house, especially in the morning, when nobody calls."

Privacy, personal space, freedom to do as you please and release from external demands, reduce tension and facilitate your personal health and centeredness. To quote Oscar Wilde, "To love oneself is the beginning of a lifelong romance." No such romance is possible if you are deprived of time and space to get to know the person within. Time alone is important because it is during these moments that you are moved toward self-reflection and introspection. The peace-rendering qualities of solitude remind you of your basic values and renew personal resources as you greet the challenges of your daily life.

INTERNAL AND EXTERNAL TIME

"Time pressures" are major stress inducers in our lives. We are behind time, we race against time, we run out of time and are squeezed by a shortage of time. We are greeted in the morning by an "alarm clock" that launches us into a time measured world, to scurry through the house, out the door, into a world getting to work on time. The workday marches on until the appointed hour. Even life at home is parceled into dinner times, bedtimes, weekends and annual vacations.

Because we are so governed by external time, time imposed on us by the clock, we forget about another kind of time: our own, unique, inner sense of time. There is a clock within, differing from person to person. One of our deepest feelings is this inner rhythm, so uniquely our own. When our inner clock ticks evenly, moderately and in concert with external time, we feel relaxed and competent. When we feel rushed and in conflict with external time, we feel distracted and tense and incompetent; our inner demands are competing with external demands.

Imagine awakening every morning without a schedule. What would you do? How would you know what to do and when to do it? This is the world our ancestors survived in; they were in touch with larger rhythms. Their basic instincts, intuitions, inner rhythms and internal clocks, played important roles as they lived in concert with unlabeled, natural time. As we became more cerebral and societal, we calibrated this unfolding process into a time binding mold; a life process now dominated by ticking clocks, appointments, and calendar dates. In so doing, we laid the groundwork for our modern, tightly scheduled way of living.

Like other living things, we too follow cycles. Our body temperature is typically at its lowest about 4:00 AM. We are more alert and productive during certain times of the day. Times of heightened and lowered appetite, sexual urge, energy level, mental alertness, and many other aspects of our personal functioning follow predictable daily cycles. When our natural inner rhythms conflict with external circumstances so often man-made, we feel uncomfortable and eventually react defiantly.

Because you have an inner clock, inner rhythms, and a uniqueness in this regard, you want to be aware of this important element of yourself. Examine yourself as you consider the following questions. Your answers will help you determine how influenced you are by internal rhythms.

Can you change your sleep schedule and still feel rested?

Can you work in the morning as well as in the evening?

Must you eat at certain times of the day, or can you vary this with changing circumstances?

Do you adjust to jet lag without discomfort?

BEING RELAXED AND IN THE ZONE

Your ability to relax is very much a matter of how your inner rhythms work together. Like a spinning top, you are most effective when your movements are effectively coordinated around a quiet center. Feelings of relaxation and self-confidence are more likely when you are rested and nutritionally balanced, and when you allow yourself to go with the process of constructive change; when you allow yourself to grow in the direction of your inner callings and coordinate your longings with the needs of those around you. This does not imply you become passive, idle, or lack initiative. It means, more than anything, your ability to place yourself fully in the midst of forward moving action, which leads us to our next key concept: balance, of things within you, with things around you.

BALANCE

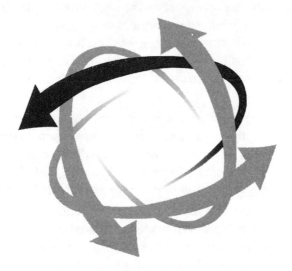

BALANCE

What's the first thought that comes to mind when you hear the word *balance*? Is it something dull but necessary, like balancing your checkbook? Something that is by definition static, motionless, neutral?

Check those thoughts at the door and open your mind to a different way of thinking about balance. Think of it first of all as dynamic — poise in action, force and counterforce in equal tension. Think of the acrobat on the high wire. Replay in your mind's eye one of those supreme moments in sports shown again and again in slow motion — Michael Jordan rising up and up for an impossible shot he's going to make, gymnast Mary Lou Retton descending from an explosive vault to nail a perfect landing.

Think of yourself at the absolute pinnacle of readiness, at the very moment of stepping off into the unknown. What is the physical feeling you want to have in that ultimate moment, the state of mind you need, to meet and master that challenge? Now you're getting closer to what we mean by balance.

This feeling of poised readiness for action involves both relaxation and balance. When we are relaxed and balanced, we are working comfortably without tension and strain. For our bodies, this means working with the force of gravity to produce movements that are coordinated, and efficient. In this chapter you'll learn to integrate your relaxed inner self with your balanced physical body. You will learn the Position of Strength. You'll learn how to stay within your Back Safety Zone and how to develop a full body attitude that uses more of your muscles to support balanced movement.

All balance requires a pivotal point. In this case, the pivotal point is within you and is called your center. So locating, recognizing, and using your center — both in body and mind —

is a crucial first step. When you function from your center, *mentally*, your actions are grounded in deeply held personal values. When you function from your center, *physically*, your actions are balanced around your body's center of gravity. In a fully balanced person, these two processes are ongoing and intimately interrelated.

Balance when internalized brings about mental stability, emotional steadiness, a continuing disposition of calm behavior, an imperturbable readiness for any change and challenge. When this centeredness is established in your mind, you can learn to communicate these qualities with balanced, coordinated physical movement. More attention to your body's habits of communication will help you to project a better image, more fully express your intentions and enhance your interpersonal dealings.

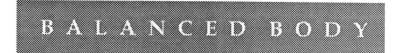

BALANCED BODY

THE BODY UPRIGHT

Every physical movement you will ever make takes place in a gravitational world. Physical forces govern your bodily movements as you work, play, lift, turn, push, pull, and so on. To be fully effective and efficient, you want to acknowledge these forces and learn to work with them. You want your physical activities to be in concert with the physical laws of nature. You want to be balanced, to maintain equilibrium, in all your daily activities.

Consider the following: only our species walks straight upright, with a forward gait. We took "verticality" on with full commitment. We gave up the stability of four-legged support for a more gravitationally compromised two-legged stance. With this exchange we gained the full use of our hands and began our history of tool use and technological advancement.

As you stand, you experience the downward pull of gravity on your body. To move with ease and grace in the vertical position, you must learn to move with, rather than against, the downward pull of gravity. Working with these forces also saves energy and decreases strains and sprains.

OUR VULNERABLE BODIES

Strains and sprains, like so many other physical ailments, are injuries we sometimes inflict on ourselves. They result, in part, from poor posture and incorrect body movements. We sit and stand improperly much of the time. We lift, push, pull, bend, reach and twist in such a manner that we strain muscles. Pain occurs as nature's way of telling us we are failing to take care of ourselves.

The human body is a highly complex system composed of many inter-related subsystems. Muscles, ligaments, organs, nerves and bone structures function in unison when they perform as they should. Changes in one part of the system create corresponding changes in others, allowing our bodies to maintain a healthy state of balance.

Think of the segments of your body as stacked boxes: head, neck, chest, abdomen, hips, legs, feet. Each segment must be balanced in relation to all other segments, or the whole stack will topple. Unlike a tower of boxes, your body moves and constantly shifts its center of gravity. Reach forward and your center of gravity changes. Your body stabilizes by activating the muscles that keep you from falling.

MUSCLES

Muscles are the body's anti-gravity devices. Without them we would be little more than motionless mass. We move when pairs of muscles work together. One muscle contracts to produce movement, while another relaxes to facilitate that movement. For example, you flex your arm as you contract your biceps and relax your triceps. You extend your arm by contracting your triceps, while relaxing your biceps. Balanced body movements are negotiated through dynamic coordination and cooperation among muscle groups and we move with efficiency and ease.

When our body is not in balance, body weight is, of course, unequally distributed. The muscles that are forced to carry the extra weight become tense and less flexible, leading to stiffness and pain. For example, when we move in an imbalanced manner, as when we walk with our head tilted forward, neck and shoulder muscles carry the load. As these muscles imitate the function of bone structures, they gradually become more inflexible. And as they become more rigid, blood flow is restricted. This decreases oxygenation of muscle cells, reduces nutrition to, and waste removal from, these same cells, ultimately causing increased muscle tension and biomechanical dysfunction. In short, muscles are in a state of imbalance and ill repair, and body movements are faulty.

WORKING WITH YOUR CEREBELLUM

Any discussion of physical balance would be incomplete without recognition of the essential role of the cerebellum. The cerebellum is a specialized structure in the brain located on both sides of the brain stem. It is the essential processor for many types of muscular coordination, including balance.

The chemical and electrical interchanges among muscles, and nerve cells occur at infinitesimally small fractions of time allowing for rapid, unconscious monitoring and adjustment of movement. Information from our sense organs — eyes, ears, nose, skin — and from sensory areas of the brain are also relayed to the cerebellum. Here these sensory inputs become part of the web of information that aids and refines cerebellar control.

While your cerebellum functions automatically and does not require assistance from your conscious mind, there is much you can do to consciously assist your physical balance. For example, if you walk a railroad track or tightrope, your cerebellum will do its best to keep you upright. When you consciously use relaxed breathing along with correct posture you work with your cerebellum to produce ever more effective, coordinated and balanced body movements.

THE SPINAL COLUMN

Our bodies are shaped as we grow. We begin life in the fetal position, in the shape of the letter "C". Later, we develop the ability to lift our head while in the lying down position. To accommodate this evolving ability, we develop an inward curve between the head and upper back. Then we crawl and gradually develop the ability to stand vertically. To accomplish this, we need another inward curve, but this time in the lower back. The unique spinal structure of human beings is shaped in the form of the letter "S": a relatively straight spine with inward curves in the neck and lower back. This dynamic spinal design delivers superior shock absorption for our two-legged walking. The curves also provide greater strength and protection against fracture.

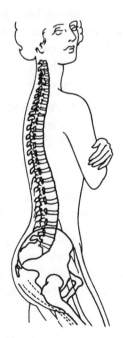

We need to maintain this wonderfully balanced spinal shape throughout the activities of daily living. When we sit, stand, or walk in slouched or unbalanced positions, we tend to look slovenly and also to strain our neck and lower back. Office workers slouched before a video display terminal, for example, tend to develop rounded shoulders and a forward head tilt. Habitually bad posture leads to health problems like muscle strains and aches. Improper body mechanics can cause damage to spinal discs.

VERTICAL EXCELLENCE

Any activity that we perform in an upright position — moving, standing, or even sitting — requires balance. We know from the study of ballet, martial arts, sports like throwing the discus, skiing, tennis, and golf, that certain conditions must be met in order to perform with excellence. Proper breathing must be coordinated with correct full body movements to achieve quickness, strength and grace.

Many athletes such as gymnasts, fencers and skaters exhibit excellent posture and balanced body movements. But there is probably no better place to learn these skills than in dance training. In *Dancing, A Guide For The Dancer You Can Be,*[1] Ellen Jacob maintains that rules of good body alignment are essentially the same for all styles of dancing. Correct posture, involves the following:

The pelvis is placed directly over the legs and the weight is carried on the whole foot. The back is long, but with a normal curve in the lower spine. The head is directly in line with the spine and the neck is long.

LIVING WITH GRAVITY

Our earliest explorations with gravity begin in the womb. Consider the perfect posture of the infant who has recently learned to sit upright. Almost invariably, head, neck and spine are perfectly aligned as the child sits up to play. And fully capable upright walking is completed so early in life that even by school age our struggles with balance are usually long forgotten.

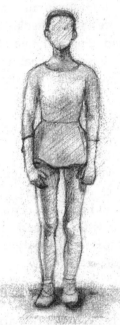

Correct Standing Posture

Though keeping our balance seems like second nature, we all know that good posture and centered action are not automatic. We can rediscover postural correctness in all our actions by becoming more consciously aware of our own body's center of gravity. We must practice operating from our center. Centeredness occurs as all the physical and mental components of our actions are totally synchronized and harmonized. We want to develop a **full body attitude**.

LOCATING YOUR CENTER THROUGH
HARD STOMACH BREATHING

Physical balance requires a center, a location around which full body movements must be coordinated for maximum effectiveness. Your center is located between your lower chest and upper thighs, in the neighborhood of your belt line. Whenever you initiate full body movements, you want to start from your center. We will do much with this concept later on as we explore full body movements in detail. For now, you want to establish a feeling of physical centeredness, which you can achieve through unification of your upper and lower body.

UNIFYING YOUR UPPER AND LOWER BODY

A good way to become aware of your physical center is through Hard Stomach Breathing. This is a simple exercise that serves to unify upper and lower abdomen creating a sensation of unity and strength.

*First, take a Soft Stomach Breath. Push your stomach out as you inhale through your nose and fill your chest with air. Hold your breath briefly, then slowly exhale through your mouth and relax. **Complete your exhalation** as you push all the air out of your body. Notice what happens: abdominal muscles contract. Upper and lower body become unified. Your physical power is more centralized.*

ON ONE FOOT

Stand up and try to balance yourself on your left foot only. Your right foot is in the air. Reach straight up with your right hand, so your arm is fully extended toward the ceiling. You are in a straightline posture at this time.

Take a deep Soft Stomach Breath and relax, allowing your body to slowly sway to the right and left. Notice how your stomach muscles automatically tighten up as you seek greater stability in this standing position. Your abdominal muscles are now coordinating your upper body movements with your lower body movements.

In this same standing position, take a deep Soft Stomach Breath and slowly exhale into a Hard Stomach Breath. Notice how conscious exhalation produces tightened abdominal muscles and enhanced physical stability. In this exercise you saw how to take conscious control over this process through Hard Stomach Breathing

HARD STOMACH BREATHING AND CENTERING

A central concept in the martial arts is that of "Ki" (pronounced *key* in Japanese), or "Chi" (*chee* in Chinese). Ki and Chi refer to the flow of energy through **the power center of your body**. Your center of power is your center of gravity, located in your lower abdomen. By unifying the upper and lower halves of your body you provide a pivot point for all full body movements.

For maximum power and coordination during full body movements, **the hips or pelvis must move first**. This is a very fundamental principle of human movement. When you move from the pelvis first, you are moving your center of gravity first, which places you in a "ready" position. (Should you move with your arms first, as you might when lifting something away from your body, you leave your center of gravity behind, and this is most cumbersome and ineffective.) Always initiate full body movements from your center and all other major body parts will automatically move with you.

THE POSITION OF WEAKNESS

Suppose you dropped a book on the floor? How would you retrieve it from a standing position?

Try this movement: Stand up with your legs straight. Bend forward at the waist and reach for something away from your body.

This most common and risky body stance is the *position of weakness*. When you move into this position, your upper body is working in opposition to your lower body, creating great stress on your lower back. This is a primary cause of back problems and a most inefficient body movement.

You need to replace this hazardous body posture with the Position of Strength, a full body posture useful for all full body

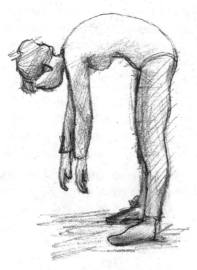

Position of Weakness

movements. In so doing, you will develop greater physical strength, quicken your body movements, protect your back and neck, and exhibit a more commanding and handsome posture.

DEVELOPING YOUR POSITION OF STRENGTH

You are now going to learn the proper stance for maintaining balance during all kinds of physical activity, from athletic competition to everyday bending and lifting. First you will learn the basic Position of Strength. Then you will practice a series of exercises for using the Position of Strength while in motion.

BASIC STEPS

You will first learn to stand correctly in the Position of Strength. Stand upright in your normal standing position. Notice your legs. Are they straight or are they bent? Most people have straight legs.

*Spread your feet so they are about shoulder width apart and **bend your knees slightly**. Your center of gravity is now closer* *to the ground and thus more stable. The lower stance also activates thigh muscles. Thigh muscles are among your body's most powerful assets. They are large and strong and you want to take advantage of them whenever you can.*

Notice your chest. Is it sort of sunken, or is it pushed way out? Neither position is correct. **Push your chest only slightly forward.** *Notice how this creates a nice inward curve in your low back.* **Allow your shoulders to fall to a natural position** *as you keep your chest in a slightly forward position.*

Exhale into a Hard Stomach Breath and notice your tightened stomach muscles. This gives you a feel for the stability and strength of your full body posture.

Your hands should be close to your body. This gives you greater quickness and power.

Take a Soft Stomach Breath and notice how good it feels. You are now relaxed and balanced in the Position of Strength.

THE POSITION OF STRENGTH KATA

Now you want to practice putting this balanced, centered posture into motion, by using the Position of Strength Kata. "Kata" (pronounced *kah-tah*) is a Japanese word meaning "form". In traditional martial arts training, katas are sequences of basic body postures and movements, practiced to perfection, eventually performed fluidly and seamlessly in sequence without conscious thought.

The Position of Strength Kata will help you practice using the Position of Strength throughout a series of different body movements. In other words, you will learn how to maintain the same body posture, regardless of what you do in the course of your day.

Read through the description of the kata sequence then practice the kata until your performance is smooth and flowing. But before you begin, here are some tips that will help you enjoy and increase the benefits of the Position of Strength Kata, or any similar exercise:

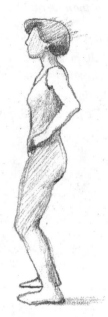

Position of Strength

Move in slow motion. *This helps you to focus on your movements and to know whether you are actually moving correctly.*

Imagine you are performing before an audience. *This activates emotional responses, adding life to your performance. Imagine, for example, as you perform the acts of standing or sitting, that you are at an important ceremony in front of royalty or dignitaries. This kind of imagining or visualization process is highly effective and frequently used by mimes, competitive athletes and many others to enhance performance.*

Imagine yourself on video*, and every once in a while freeze the frame. Stop whatever you are doing and study your posture. Go from slow motion to no motion and see what happens. Use a mirror if available. Better yet, if you have video recording equipment, use it. You might be amazed to see how you really* *look*—*as opposed to how you think you look. Remember, body language speaks louder than words.*

Step 1: Lie Down in the Position of Comfort

With your chest slightly forward, drop to one knee, then onto your shoulder. Roll onto your back into the lying down position.

Bring your knees into the bent knee position as you enter the Position of Comfort. Do three Soft Stomach Breaths and relax.

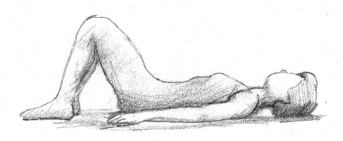

Position of Comfort

Step 2: Rise to the Position of Strength

Roll onto your shoulder, then rise to one knee. Push your chest slightly forward and rise to a standing position.

Step 3: Stand in the Position of Strength

With your feet shoulder width apart, push your chest forward and bend your knees slightly. You are in the Position of Strength.

Take a Soft Stomach Breath and relax. Take another Soft Stomach Breath and slowly exhale as you relax your face, shoulders and body down through your thighs. Your knees should be slightly bent.

Come up onto your toes, then back down and center your weight over the arches of your feet.

*You are **relaxed and balanced** in the Position of Strength. Notice how your weight is felt most in your buttocks, lower legs* *and feet. Balance occurs when your body weight is equally distributed over your base of support.*

Step 4: Combining Soft and Hard Stomach Breathing

Take a Soft Stomach Breath and slowly exhale into a Hard Stomach Breath and notice your stomach muscles tighten.

Your lower abdomen now feels connected to the feeling you experience as you balance your weight over your arches.

Step 5: Reaching in the Position of Strength

*To reach correctly in the Position of Strength, you will need to be aware of your **Back Safety Zone**. Imagine a cylinder around your body. Point your elbow in front of you. The area from your chest to your elbow, is your Back Safety Zone. It is also your zone of maximum physical power.*

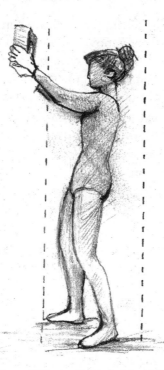

Reaching in Position of Strength Outside of Back Safety Zone

When you use the Position of Strength, within your Back Safety Zone, you are protecting yourself from injury and are increasing physical power. Not a bad combination.

Imagine you are in The Position of Strength, reaching for a heavy box on a shelf slightly above your shoulders. Maintain the Position of Strength and exhale into the exertion as you reach. Quickly bring the box into your Back Safety Zone.

Think of something you do during the day that causes you to reach outside your Back Safety Zone, leading you into the Position of Weakness. Reaching for golf clubs in the trunk of your car, or for a baby in a crib, are good examples. A mechanic changing spark plugs, reaching over the engine, and exerting himself in the Position of Weakness is another.

PIVOTING IN THE POSITION OF STRENGTH

Very high risk of injury occurs when you **twist at the waist;** your upper body moves in one direction as your lower body moves in the other. If, for example, you twist while lifting boxes from a stack on your left to a stack on your right, you are on your way to developing a major back problem.

The proper way to turn from one direction to another, is to **pivot in the position of strength**: your shoulders and hips move together as one foot remains in place, and the other moves into the new direction.

Imagine holding a basketball. Basketball players keep a wide base of support for stability in the Position of Strength. (This is equally true of tennis, wrestling, badminton, racquetball and most other sports.)

Pivot to face someone on your left who is throwing the ball to you.

Catch the ball. Exhale as you pivot and throw the ball to someone on your right.

Pivot to the left to receive another ball. Pivot to the right and exhale as you throw it once again.

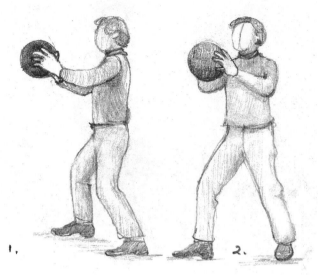

Pivoting in Position of Strength

SITTING IN THE POSITION OF STRENGTH

Find a chair and sit down. Slouch into the chair as you gradually yield to the downward pull of gravity. Now sit properly. Bring your chest forward, and position your head directly over your shoulders. This produces a nice inward curve in your lower back. You are now sitting in the Position of Strength.

Frequent slouching in the sitting position causes neck and low back strain. Acquiring correct sitting habits requires concentration. When you sit, you probably forget about your posture, because you are focused on other things like reading or watching television.

THE POSITION OF STRENGTH IN SPORTS AND DANCE

You want to use the posture of the Position of Strength throughout all your full body movements. You want to be

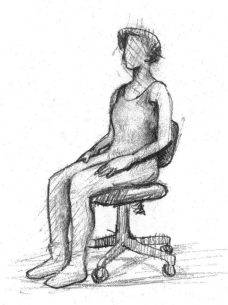

Sitting in Position of Strength

vertical and to move from the pelvis first. Such relaxed full body movements are graceful, energy-efficient, quick and powerful.

A scene in a wonderful old Japanese movie called *The Seven Samurai*[2] vividly illustrates the power and significance of a balanced full body attitude. A group of Japanese farmers is searching for skilled warriors to protect them from brigands who annually pillage their village. In their search, they hear of a samurai working nearby, chopping wood in exchange for food.

The scene introducing the samurai shows him chopping wood with a perfectly straight back, knees bent, exhaling into the exertion. Although correct wood chopping technique may be of little interest to the beleaguered farmers, not to mention the movie's audience, it is of considerable relevance to the samurai's capabilities, and to the authenticity of the actor's performance. Any deviation from centered, balanced action would be readily observed by a trained eye, revealing whether this samurai is authentic or not.

SUMO WRESTLING

Sumo is Japan's national sport. Competitive events typically last less than a minute. After a series of limbering-up exercises and ceremonial acts, the two wrestlers face each other in the center of the ring, assuming an aggressive crouch position. On the referee's signal, they charge and meet with an awesome smack. This is the moment of truth in Sumo.

Sumo wrestlers always maintain the Position of Strength. The key to their great strength is in their legs and hips. The basic aim of their approach to body-building is to create a low center of gravity for balance and stability. As in all forms of wrestling, functioning from your center is critical to balance, stability and strength.

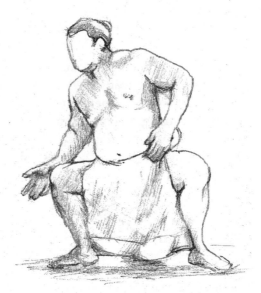

Sumo Wrestlers Create A Low Center of Gravity

The inexperienced observer of Sumo wrestlers may assume that because of their large, protruding bellies they are fat and not in the best of shape. In fact, the ideal Sumo wrestler's body has extensive muscle development with a thin layer of fat. The protruding belly is said to be as strong as a brick wall.

There is hardly a better example of physical centeredness than that provided by the skilled Sumo wrestler. It is interesting to note that their great balance and power resulting from stance and posture enable Sumo wrestlers to pick up such sports as surfing with relative ease. Their agility and balance is particularly impressive, considering their physical size and bulk.

JUDO

Judo requires balancing your own body while unbalancing the body of the opponent. The natural stance of Judo is one of the keys to effectiveness in this sport. Correct stance involves facing the opponent with weight equally distributed and legs spread slightly apart. Back is straight, arms hang loosely at the side, with relaxed shoulders and knees. Judo provides another excellent example of the Position of Strength in action.

Someone trained in Judo has a distinctive walk. They move with feet spread slightly apart, weight is equally distributed, knees are slightly bent and movement comes from the hips and the abdomen where strength comes from. Peak performing athletes always **move from the pelvis first**. As in other activities like football and baseball, proper stance delivers balance, coordination, power and the best results. The principle for proper stance is to **bend your knees**, which lowers your center of gravity and facilitates balance and stability.

Think of your body in the shape of a triangle, with your head at the top and feet at the bottom two points, about shoulder width apart. Draw a straight line from the top of your head to the base of the triangle. The line will pass through your center of gravity, ending midway between your feet. In oriental cultures, a triangular posture is evidence of strength and stability.

In occidental cultures, emphasis is often on size and strength of upper body muscles, suggestive of an inverted triangle or top. But in the presence of gravity, the triangle with its base down is a much more stable shape.

BALLET AND TAI-CHI

Ballet training produces excellence of posture: the back long, with a nice inward curve in the lower back, the pelvis directly over the legs. Strength from abdominal and thigh muscles is critical to success. A good illustration of the Position of Strength in ballet is the pirouette, a spin usually 360 degrees or more, with the weight of the body on one foot only. The head, body and supporting leg form a vertical line. This is about as close to a "spinning top" as is humanly possible. The legs move freely around their axis, the hips. The torso does the same.

It has been said that ballet, when competently taught, is probably the best head-to-toe training system there is. It is full body exercise, with a relaxed, balanced, full body attitude. Once again, center of gravity plays a determining role. You always benefit when you function from your center.

The posture and gestures in a pirouette are similar to those used while moving from the waist in Tai-Chi. As Y.K. Chen says:

> In the waist, not the limbs, lies the mainspring of the movements of our body. The movements of the limbs are slow and short, while those of the waist are free and long. One turning of a big axis is equivalent to hundreds of turnings of small axes. The waist is similar to a big axis, and the limbs, palms, elbows, shoulders, legs, knees, heels, etc., are similar to small axes. [3]

BOWLING

Perhaps the biggest mistake made by beginning bowlers is to lean forward and muscle the ball, rather then using proper body mechanics combined with correct breathing. Use of the Position of Strength, in conjunction with correct breathing, is the proper technique.

The starting position is that of the Position of Strength, which is back straight, knees bent, with the ball close to your waist. As you move forward and release the ball, your body should be balanced on the lead foot and you should remain in the Position of Strength. Release of the ball should be fully coordinated with Exhaling Into The Exertion.

DOWNHILL SKIING

Correct downhill skiing technique illustrates the same principles of good posture. Your back is straight, feet are apart and body weight is equally distributed over both skis. Note that in skiing as in wrestling, the shoulders are rounded forward somewhat. Of course, your knees are flexed.

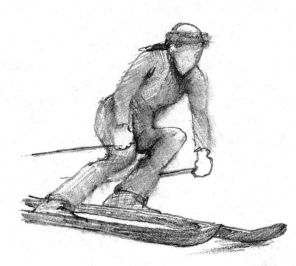

Skiier Uses Bent Knees for Stability

Jean-Claude Killy, discussing how to recover in unexpected and difficult skiing situations, declares it is most important to stay relaxed. Here he describes his technique for keeping his balance under pressure:

I was almost knocked off-balance. Just in the nick of time I recovered by doing several things simultaneously. First, I dropped my hips very low (lowered my center of gravity), put my feet farther apart, and spread my arms a bit to make sure of my stability.[4]

HORSEBACK RIDING

We have already seen how essential relaxed breathing is to what Sally Swift calls Centered Riding. She also emphasizes correct body posture. In centered riding, the rider must be physically balanced to eliminate unnecessary physical strain and tension, and to conserve energy for other uses.

To better understand physical balance, Swift divides the body into four building blocks: head and neck; rib cage and shoulders; pelvis; legs and feet. These four body areas must be properly aligned and balanced. Again, we see the importance of the Position of Strength: back is straight, knees are slightly bent.

The basic principle, applied to all correct riding positions, is to maintain your center of gravity over your feet at all times. When galloping or jumping, for example, the rider leans forward to maintain balance. Forward weight of the upper body is balanced by the weight of the hips, while the center of gravity remains over the feet. Once again, the key is to function from the center at all times.

GOLF

Excellence of golf technique is highly dependent on physical balance and coordinated full body movements. Throughout the swing, it is important to maintain proper balance so your swing is coordinated with your center of gravity. Your shoulders, waist and knees must maintain full body coordination, or they will compete with each other, reducing power. Golf is an excellent example of the importance of relaxed, balanced, full body movements in the Position of Strength.

BALANCED MIND

INTERNALIZING BALANCE

These sports are by no means the only ones where principles of balance come into play. If there's a sport or physical activity that you engage in regularly that has not been mentioned, you can analyze for yourself the correct posture and stance to use. It might even make a humdrum routine more interesting: carrying groceries, mowing the lawn, picking up a child, standing on a moving bus or subway car. Practicing the Position of Strength Kata should help you to internalize relaxed full body movement, so that it becomes second nature.

Be guided also by the information you have learned in this chapter: use Hard Stomach Breathing, move from the pelvis, stay within your Back Safety Zone, lower your stance for greater stability, use thigh muscles for additional power. Perhaps most important of all, concentrate on the feeling of strength and stability that suffuses your mind when you engage in full body movements in the Position of Strength.

This body/mind sensation can become a valuable resource, one you can use in the face of challenging situations of all types, whenever you need to "get a grip". With practice you will be able to bring about a steady and strong mental state and dispel negative, unsettling emotions by calling to mind this feeling of centeredness.

The route to that centered feeling will be different for different people. For some, the memory of the body/mind sensation may be enough. Taking a hard stomach breath may work as a trigger. Perhaps you'll need a verbal message or mental image or maybe a combination of things. It's worth some time and effort to arrive at a simple way for you to do this.

Try the following exercise with a partner. It may help you to arrive at a particular route to your mental Position of Strength.

Imagine that your center is not at your physical center of gravity, but is instead in the middle of your forehead. You might try touching that spot to focus your attention there, or visualizing a symbol for your center and mentally placing it in the middle of your forehead. (This symbol could be a word or an image, for example a target, or concentric circles or spokes of a wheel around a midpoint.)

Close your eyes, concentrating on this center in the middle of your forehead. Have your partner try to push you off balance by shoving gently but firmly against your shoulder.

How easily were you able to maintain your balance? Did you notice how you automatically tightened your stomach muscles for support?

Try again. Assume a comfortable, relaxed standing position. This time imagine that your center of gravity is in your abdomen. Locate your center with a Hard Stomach Breath and mentally focus on your body's real center of gravity. (Once again, it may help you to mentally "see" some symbol of balance or strength as occupying this place in your lower abdomen.)

How did this experience differ from the previous one? Try reversing roles with your partner.

BREATHING AND BALANCE

Now try this exercise:

Stand fully upright with your chest slightly forward. Place one foot directly in front of the other so they are in a straight line. The toe of one foot is touching the heel of the other.

Imagine you are walking a tightrope. Extend your arms out to your sides and balance yourself in each of two ways:

First, balance yourself as you take a few Soft Stomach Breaths. Notice how physical relaxation facilitates balance.

Now, focus attention on your physical center of gravity and balance across the tightrope. Inhale with a Soft Stomach Breath as you begin to move the back foot to the front and exhale into a Hard Stomach Breath as you set your foot down in the forward position.

You are walking with perfect posture as you coordinate breathing and full body movement.

Self-confidence and strength are the result of a relaxed and balanced mind. You can attain these characteristics as you improve your physical movements and control your mental climate. These breathing and centering principles have a wide range of applications. Use them to gain composure in stressful situations, to perfect your golf game, to mentally prepare for a challenging task. These activities are beneficial in all your dealings because they enable you to work from your center.

INTEGRITY, INNER BALANCE AND CENTEREDNESS

When physical, mental and emotional aspects of our being are integrated and balanced in our actions, we are centered. In the absence of this guiding force, we are a ship at sea, with damaged rudder and no reliable sense of direction.

Integrity can be viewed from many perspectives. It is a gyroscope within, our moral equilibrium, ability to decipher right from wrong, fairness from unfairness, straightforwardness from deviousness. It is a constant that lies at the base of our moral decisions. It is knowing we are what we do, and we do what is right, to the best of our ability.

We sense our own integrity through inner balance and feelings of centeredness. It is an inner calmness, dramatically evident in our actions. In archery, an arrow correctly released, flies straight and true. Personal integrity is a straight line force, that helps us express ourselves with clarity, decisiveness, consistency, and credibility. When we sense integrity in others, we feel their strength and trust their motives. It is everything about us that determines the value of our handshake. It can be gained and it can be lost. It all depends on what we do and how we live our lives.

The true test of integrity takes place over time. Integrity requires we know ourselves and behave in accordance with our beliefs; we stand behind them when they are valid and discard them when they are not. Integrity, by its very nature, requires us to change as we encounter new and better ways to view the world. Desire to forge principles and beliefs that stand the test of time lies at the very basis of this noblest of human qualities.

USING BODY LANGUAGE TO EXPRESS YOUR INTEGRITY

Actions, we all know, speak louder than words, and when it comes to conveying who you really are, your body speaks loud and clear, whether you intend it or not. The Position of Strength is an excellent example. It speaks for you with considerable authority. You look and act more confidently, because you are in a better position to do so.

Most of the really important things you do in life involve other people. Your skill and ease with people, your ability to lead, depends very much on your physical expression. If you want to make a positive, strong impression, to have people truly understand you and everything you stand for, you need to perfect your body language so that it really expresses your internal workings, your integrity and wholeness.

With this in mind, there is a lot you can learn from some of the most articulate practitioners of body language, the masters of mime. In the words of the greatest of them all, Marcel Marceau, "The most important feeling in life is self-command. This is the only way to lead men to rule over their passion and reach the most precious aim in life, liberty."[5]

Mime is the ultimate in body language. It is communication by physical posture, gesture and expression. Becoming a mime involves a great deal of body training. Mimes must be aware of each separate body component. As in dance training, emphasis is on balanced verticality of head, neck, shoulders, diaphragm, ribs, stomach, thighs and feet. Control of each of these body components is essential to the creation of different mime effects.

Mimes must be keenly attuned to the human vocabulary of emotion. They must be able to physically express internal states of mind. They must match their audience's great skill at understanding body language. We are able to understand the feelings, motives and characters of other people mainly through gestures, postures and facial expressions. People routinely make negative appraisals of character and competence when they sense nervousness, indecisiveness, sloppiness, belligerence or other indications of mental disequilibrium. You have probably made some of these judgements yourself.

You may be an expert in reading body language. But are you fully in control of your own physical expression? What kind of image do you project? Are you communicating relaxed strength and equilibrium? You already know how to calm yourself through relaxed Soft Stomach Breathing and how to strengthen your resolve with the Position of Strength. Now we suggest that you explore your control of body language with some basic mime exercises.

THE DOUBLE-ZERO POSITION

Try the basic mime position, the Double-Zero Position.

Stand erect with heels together and feet at a ninety degree angle.

Push your chest forward and lengthen your neck so it is in a straight line position. Relax your arms and keep your legs straight. This is the Double-Zero Position and the normal standing position for a mime.

Soft Stomach Breathing is also essential to mime technique. To maintain a "position of silence", it is important the chest not move and this is possible only through Soft Stomach Breathing.

The Double-Zero is quite "expressionless." It's like a blank slate on which anything may be written. Imagine yourself in this position and visualize how you might add some personality to your appearance. You can add pleasing effects or you can add displeasing effects.

Assume the Double-Zero position. Now create a personality that appears tired, withdrawn, and burned out. Drop your head, let your shoulders fall into a slouch, let your chest sink in, and round your back. For greater effect, extend your lower lip and

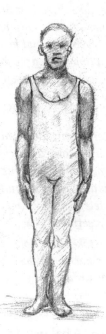

The Double Zero Position

create a long, drawn out, facial expression. A vacant stare will accent the overall effect.

Leave this weary appearance behind and develop a more lively, energetic personality. Lift your head, push your chest forward, which brings your shoulders into proper position, as it also creates a nice inward curve in your low back. Smile with your lips and eyes. Quite a difference, wouldn't you agree?

TENSION VERSUS RELAXATION

Stand in the Double-Zero position. Tighten your entire body so all your muscles feel rigid. Widen your eyes and look totally frightened. Imagine you are in the office of your boss, who is about to fire you because of your overall incompetence. You are now a good example of someone lacking in self-confidence and full of fear.

To change this attitude, take three Soft Stomach Breaths, relax all of your muscles throughout your body. Pay particular attention to your eyes, eyebrows and facial muscles. Imagine you are receiving a compliment for a job well done. You are now a good example of a self-confident person with no visible fears.

ANGER VERSUS JOY

Stand in the Double-Zero position. Tighten your jaw muscles, your fists, and stomach muscles. Imagine you are stopped in heavy traffic. Every time your car begins to move, you quickly come to a halt. Traffic is at a standstill and you are trapped. You have no way to make a telephone call and you are worried about missing an important meeting,

To change this attitude, take three Soft Stomach Breaths, relax your jaw, fists, and stomach muscles. Imagine you are on a Hawaiian beach with your favorite person. Your life is perfect and you just received news of your award for best person of the year. A smile creeps over your face and you want to jump for joy.

It's simple and clear. A balanced and relaxed appearance projects positive, steady qualities. Communicating inner strength is a matter of consciously controlling your physical and mental state through Soft Stomach Breathing and balanced posture, particularly the Position of Strength.

When you are balanced and centered, you feel integrated, self-directed, in concert with yourself and your surroundings. You can more readily make choices and decisions, and know the direction you want to go. You are always acting from a Position of Strength, because your Position of Strength moves as you move.

Just as a mime is free and ready to take on any role and posture from the Double-Zero position, when you are truly in balance you are primed to move in any direction and act in any situation. Balance is the starting point for any action — mental or physical — and the key to successful completion of that action.

FLEXIBILITY

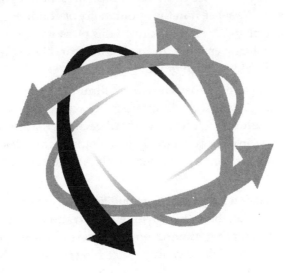

FLEXIBILITY

What is more malleable is always superior over that which is immovable. This is the principle of controlling things by going along with them, of mastery through adaptation.

— Lao-Tzu[1]

Joy in movement! It is a free and flowing embodiment of living energy. We see it in the suppleness of a gymnast's movement. We sense it in the spontaneity of children's rough and tumble play. We have all known this pleasurable sensation. We feel it whenever body and mind inseparably express the freedom, the aliveness of movement.

Tension and stiffness however, diminish the pleasure in movement. You need flexibility to move with ease. Touching your toes, turning your head, without back pain, without neck pain — you can only move freely when muscles are elastic and joints are limber. Perhaps it's been a while since you've felt this way.

No matter what your age or condition, you can dramatically increase your flexibility by learning how to stretch. Stretching brings on a liberating, energizing sensation that makes you feel good, makes you radiate vitality. Stretching moves you beyond limitations, allows you to do what you could not do before. Stretching extends your reach in both body and mind.

First you will explore the physical aspects of flexibility. You will learn to stretch and begin to limber up muscles and move again. Maybe you'll be able to do some things you haven't tried for many years.

Then we'll look inward to the expansive, empowering sensations of mental flexibility too. I can't overstate the importance of flexibility when it comes to problem-solving and inter-personal dealings. Breakthroughs, in personal relationships and in professional life do not arise by trying harder with the same means and plans. Progress, innovations, solutions, resolutions require flexibility to some degree. You can practice flexibility and improve your physical and mental ability to stretch.

FLEXIBLE BODY

As skyscrapers yield to high winds and earthquakes, so do flexible people greet challenge and change. Freedom of movement, the ability to take alternate courses of action, is essential to a state of readiness, important for both physical and mental performance. Flexibility, when integrated with relaxation and balance skills, facilitates our readiness for action.

You already have some experience with relaxation and balance. Flexibility is really an extension and development of these. To maintain flexibility, muscles must be relaxed and must be used in balanced ways.

Injury to muscle from overwork, strain, tension, leads to sustained shortening of muscle fibers. Aging and lack of exercise can have the same effects. Muscle shortening causes tightness and interferes with the range and the fluidity of your movements.

Chronically shortened muscles have diminished power as well. They can do less work because their ability to contract is limited. If you examine how muscle fibers operate you can see why this is true.

THE SECRET LIFE OF MUSCLES

The secret of muscle power lies in the unique construction of muscle cells. Here design is perfectly suited to the task of the cell: contraction. Each muscle cell is comprised of smaller strands of fibers called myofibrils. A cell may have hundreds to thousands of these smaller strands.

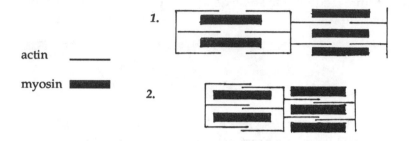

actin _____

myosin ███████

Diagram of Muscle Proteins (1. rest state, 2. contracted)

Myofibrils are largely made of two kinds of protein, a thick protein called myosin and a thin protein called actin. These proteins are arranged in a specific pattern of alternating bands. When viewed through a microscope, muscles actually have a striped appearance because of this arrangement. Roughly speaking, areas with the thicker protein are darker in color, areas with thinner protein are lighter.

When the muscle fibers receive the signal to contract, the protein bands overlap. Specifically, actin filaments in a band of thin protein slide into the spaces between myosin filaments in a thick band. The resulting overlap causes the myofibril to shorten in length. Myofibrils acting in concert contract the muscle and produce movement. The greater the overlap of proteins, the greater the contraction. A relaxed muscle at resting state has the greatest potential for producing movement. Muscles can be restored to a proper resting state through lengthening by correct stretching exercises.

FLEXIBLE MOVEMENTS

When your muscles tighten over time from sustained tension, overuse, or disuse, your ability to move freely lessens, and you are more prone to problems like neck, shoulder, and back pain. And, as you feel increasingly restricted, you naturally lower your overall level of physical activity. You began to feel old and ever so gradually enter the sedentary life. You are less active, gain weight, have less energy, are more irritable, and generally less happy. If indeed, you are what you do, then you may become less and less as time goes on.

Without proper exercise, which includes regular stretching, muscles shorten. They accumulate waste products. Blood flow and oxygen supply to muscles diminishes. You become increasingly impaired as time goes on. When you consider that about 42 percent of male body weight and 36 percent of female body weight is skeletal muscle tissue, it is easy to see why it is so important to keep your muscles in a healthy, flexible state of repair.

We are conscious of our muscles primarily through aches, pains and overall tightness. The older we get, the more this seems to be true. We marvel at children and how they move about with such elasticity and freedom, and assume this is something only for the young. This is untrue. Flexibility can be acquired at any time in your life. The first step is to **become more aware** of your tensions and tight muscles.

SELF-EXPLORATION

Becoming aware of your muscle tightness is quite simple. Move almost any part of your body and you will sense whatever restriction is there. Try the following:

Slowly reach toward the ceiling. Bring your arms slowly down to your sides and notice any feeling of tightness. You may feel this somewhere deeply within your shoulders, in the back of your arms, around the base of the neck.

Most of us are fairly tight throughout our neck, shoulders and upper back because we do little or nothing to alter the situation. For example, we will type for hours in a strained sitting position and rarely think of stretching. If we do, we may not know how to stretch correctly.

STRETCHING

Have you noticed how people who have been sitting for a long time, stand up and bend backwards? It is as if they know, deep down, this is good for them. They are like cats who wake from sleep, stretch every inch of their body and then move on, ready for action. Cats know what to do instinctively, and stretch frequently as a matter of course.

Stretching is the way that cats and humans lengthen their muscles and tendons. While humans also have a natural inclination to stretch, we have to first learn how to stretch correctly and then discipline ourselves to stretch on a regular basis. This requires effort at first, but the positive feelings and renewed physical capabilities that accompany regular stretching are worth the effort.

YOGA AND TAI CHI

Asian cultures which have traditionally embraced the unity of body and mind, have well-developed physical regimens that stretch the whole body.

Yoga is an ancient Hindu practice for the development of the total person and widely practiced throughout the world to this day. It involves mental and physical discipline in the pursuit of health and clarity of mind. Through correct breathing and relaxation, correct body postures, stretching and strengthening exercises, Yoga Masters achieve high levels of physical proficiency.

Yoga practice begins with the recognition of the importance of relaxation:

> Before learning any physical or mental exercise one should first learn to observe and be aware of muscular tension and be able to relax unnecessary tension of the muscles.[2]

In the practice of Yoga, emphasis is on breathing skills essential to full body relaxation, body postures conducive to full body balance, and flexible body movements that exercise and stretch the entire body.

Tai Chi, developed originally by the Chinese, is also a form of full body exercise. It begins with fundamental principles similar to Yoga:

*The body must be **comfortable** which means without tension and force, as discussed in Relaxation.*

*The body must be **vertical** which means not to lean (e.g., Position of Weakness) and must function as a single unit, as discussed in Balance.*

Tai Chi is performed slowly, gracefully, with calm physical movements. It is like a beautiful dance in slow motion. It is difficult to observe what Tai Chi "is" because most of what happens occurs within the person doing it. The basic Tai Chi standing position is described in *Tai Chi, A Way of Centering and I Ching*:

> The body is naturally erect, feet apart as wide as shoulders, parallel to each other, with toes pointing straight ahead. The center of gravity is between the two feet. Both hands drop naturally to the sides. Eyes look straight ahead. The whole body is loose and breathing naturally.[3]

Both Yoga and Tai Chi are excellent physical disciplines to stretch and tone the body and improve mental outlook. For most of us, however, it is impractical to become fully committed practitioners of Tai Chi or Yoga.

EIGHT PRINCIPLES OF CORRECT STRETCHING

The practical solution is to learn relaxed stretching exercises involving full body movements guided by a full body attitude. The stretching exercises we offer here will emphasize deliberate relaxation of muscles and balanced body movements. So you will learn to coordinate breathing with movements to facilitate full body stretching.

The following principles for effective stretching will assist you in your development of an effective stretching routine:

Principle One: It is better not to stretch at all than to stretch incorrectly. Incorrect stretching causes considerable harm to your muscles, ligaments and spine.

Principle Two: Stretching is a gentle and relaxed process. When possible, stretch in a quiet place with few distractions. Relaxed concentration is the key.

Principle Three: Correct breathing must be coordinated with correct stretching technique. Integrate Soft Stomach Breathing with your stretches. This facilitates a relaxed stretching style.

Principle Four: If stretching causes pain, STOP! Stretch only to the point of mild tension. If you stretch beyond this point, for example until you feel pain, a reflex is activated which contracts your muscles.

Principle Five: Do each stretch three times, holding each stretch a little longer then the previous one. Begin your stretches by holding about 5 seconds to evaluate your condition. If no pain occurs, then hold for up to 30 seconds on the second and third stretches.

Principle Six: Warm-up exercises get the muscles working and bring warm, oxygenated blood to the areas to be stretched. This reduces likelihood of injury and facilitates overall ease of stretching. Warm-up exercises also bring body fluids to the joints. Since major joints (i.e., elbows, knees) tend to stiffen somewhat following inactivity, warm-up exercises are beneficial for joints as well as for muscles.

Principle Seven: Stretch frequently throughout the day. Muscles tighten as the day wears on. Learn stretches that can be done in work clothes.

Principle Eight: Stretch to feel good. You will feel better as you become more flexible.

WHEN IS STRETCHING INCORRECT?

To experience how it feels to stretch incorrectly, perform the following exercise. You will quickly see how incorrect breathing interferes with stretching.

Enter the Position of Comfort. Take a deep Soft Stomach Breath and "hold it" and then bring both knees to your chest. Notice how uncomfortable you are. This is "incorrect" procedure and stretching exercises do not work when you hold your breath.

Now, for contrast, try doing the same thing *correctly*:

You are in the Position of Comfort. Take a Soft Stomach Breath and "slowly exhale" as you bring both knees to your chest. See how much easier this is? As you exhale, you relax into the stretch. Repeat this stretch a few more times and see how stretching feels good when done correctly.

STRETCHING ROUTINE WHILE LYING DOWN

DEEP BREATHING IN THE POSITION OF COMFORT
(RELAXES THE ENTIRE BODY)

Lie on your back with knees bent and arms resting at your sides or lightly on your stomach. Tighten stomach and buttock muscles and push your back against the floor. Then "inhale" to the count of four with a Soft Stomach Breath and slowly "exhale" to the count of eight. Repeat this three times.

ONE KNEE TO CHEST (STRETCHES LOWER BACK)

You are in the Position of Comfort. Inhale deeply then slowly exhale as you gently bring one knee to your chest, keeping your low back flat and head on the floor. Hold the stretch position for five seconds. Inhale with a Soft Stomach Breath and then slowly exhale as you return your leg to the bent knee position. Do the same with the other leg. Repeat this three times.

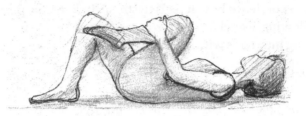

One Knee to Chest

BOTH KNEES TO CHEST (STRETCHES LOWER BACK)

You are in the Position of Comfort. Take a deep breath as you place both hands in front of your knees. Slowly exhale as you pull your knees to your chest, keeping your head on the floor. Hold for a few seconds. Return to the Position of Comfort and relax. Repeat this three times.

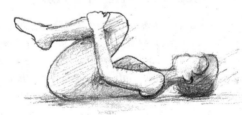

Both Knees to Chest

Note: If this stretch causes pain in the center of your low back, STOP! You may have a bulging disc, requiring professional attention. If you can do this stretch without pain, proceed to the next stretch.

HAMSTRING STRETCH
(STRETCHES MUSCLES ALONG THE BACKS OF YOUR LEGS)

In the Position of Comfort, take a deep breath and exhale as you gradually bring one knee to your chest. Slowly, extend your leg upward to the point of mild tension and hold. Make sure your toes are flexed toward your head, not the ceiling, and your head

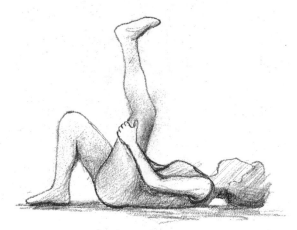

Hamstring Stretch

is on the floor. HOLD. Gradually bend your leg and inhale as you return to the Position of Comfort. Repeat the same procedure with the other leg. Do this three times.

STRETCHING ROUTINE WHILE SITTING

HEAD ROLL (STRETCHES NECK MUSCLES)

Sit in the Position of Strength. Take a deep breath and exhale as you drop your chin toward your chest. Slowly roll your head so your ear is leaning toward your shoulder. Relax and hold. Roll your head to the center and lift your chin straight up. (Do not roll your head in a circle or you may compress the bony protuberances at the back of your head.) Slowly inhale and repeat to the other side. Repeat this three times.

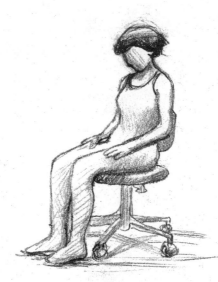

Head Roll

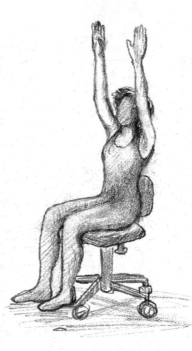

Upward Reach

UPWARD REACH
(STRETCHES UPPER BACK, SHOULDERS AND NECK)

Sit in the Position of Strength, which means you have a straight back with a nice inward curve in your low back. Inhale, and slowly exhale as you reach to the ceiling. Then slowly drop your hands down to your sides. Do this three times.

SHOULDER BLADE SQUEEZE
(STRETCHES UPPER BACK, SHOULDERS AND ARMS)

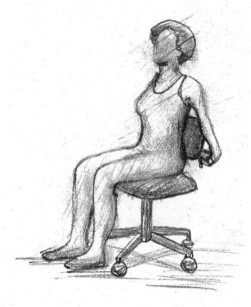

Shoulder Blade Squeeze

Sit in the Position of Strength. Reach behind your back and clasp your hands. Take a deep Soft Stomach Breath and slowly exhale as you squeeze your shoulders together (toward the center of your back) as you push your chest slightly forward and straighten your arms. Do this three times.

FORWARD BEND

(STRETCHES LOWER BACK, NECK AND SHOULDERS)

Sit forward in your chair so some weight is on your feet and legs. Spread your feet shoulder width apart. Inhale and then slowly exhale as you bend at the waist toward the floor. Drop your chin, arms and shoulders, and hang loosely for about 5 seconds.

When you have had a good stretch, tighten your stomach muscles (this supports your low back as you ascend), place your hands on your knees, and slowly exhale as you push with your hands (this takes pressure off your lower back muscles) and return to the upright position.

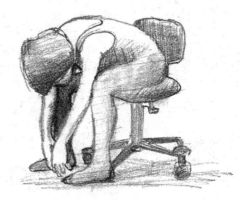

Forward Bend

STRETCHING ROUTINE WHILE STANDING

BACKWARD BEND

Stand in the Position of Strength with your chest slightly forward and knees slightly bent. Take a deep Soft Stomach Breath, slowly exhale and relax in the Position of Strength.

Take a Soft Stomach Breath as you place your hands on the small of your back and slowly exhale as you bend backward. Keep your eyes focused straight ahead and your chin on your chest to prevent tilting your head backward. Repeat three times.

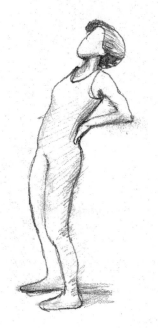

Backward Bend

UPWARD REACH

Inhale deeply as you reach for the ceiling with both arms. Exhale as you slowly drop your hands to your sides. Repeat three times.

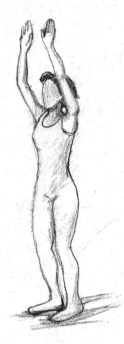

Upward Reach

STANDING HAMSTRING STRETCH

CAUTION: Do not do this stretch if you have active back pain.

Stand in the Position of Strength with knees bent. Slowly bend forward at the waist, as you let your head, shoulders and arms roll forward toward the floor. Keep your knees slightly bent as you stretch in a relaxed, comfortable manner. Take a Soft Stomach Breath and relax into the stretch as you slowly exhale.

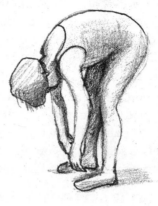

Standing Hamstring Stretch

When you feel you have had a good stretch, bend your knees, **push with your hands on your knees,** *straighten your back and slowly rise to the Position of Strength.*

CAUTION: Be absolutely certain you bend your knees as you enter and exit the stretch position.

Learning to stretch correctly is the first step. The second step requires you stretch on a regular basis. This means you must have a method of stretching that fits into your daily routine.

BRING STRETCHING INTO YOUR DAILY ROUTINE

As a general rule, you should stretch at least once a day for maintenance. Additionally, empirical evidence suggests that stretching at least twice a day is preferable. The best times appear to be in the morning after awakening (to eliminate morning stiffness and energize oneself) and in the afternoon or early evening after the day's work. However, the best time to stretch is when you feel as if you want to.[4]

Anytime you feel tension, do stretches that relieve the tightness. For example, if your job involves a good deal of sitting, stand up occasionally and do a backward bend. If your neck and shoulders are tight, do a shoulder squeeze or any movement that brings relaxation and physical activity to that area. Remember, oxygen is the life force of muscle tissue and relaxed muscles allow for necessary blood circulation.

If you are able to wear loosely fitting clothing, you will be inclined to stretch more frequently. Jeans, for example, make it difficult to do full body, hamstring stretches which are very important. Low back pain is frequently associated with tight hamstrings and this is something you can counteract through the standing hamstring stretch described earlier.

DON'T DELAY GETTING THE BENEFITS

The more you become aware of your physical tensions (i.e., head pain, neck pain, shoulder pain, low back pain) and the more you do something constructive about them, the more you progress toward self-management of your health. If you want to be flexible in your movements and pain free, increase awareness of muscle tightness and stretch frequently throughout your day.

The common belief that getting older necessarily involves severe limitations in flexibility is just not true. What we have left in our lives is time, and we want to make that time as rewarding as possible. There can be little doubt that flexibility exercises can do much to achieve this result. For example, consider signing up for a beginning Yoga class. Most communities now have these classes available in a variety of settings. Relaxed, balanced, flexible movement can make a tremendous difference in your life. Remember, you are what you do, and the more you engage in flexible, full body movements, the more effective you become in all aspects of your being.

SPORTS APPLICATIONS

Of course, if you engage in sports, competitively or recreationally, you probably know that stretching should be a regular part of your readiness preparations. Unfortunately, this does not seem to be widely enough known among children. Physical education teachers and team coaches for even the youngest children have a great opportunity in this area. They can help children form life-long habits that will help them not only in sports, but in maintaining health and vitality, physical and mental, throughout their lives.

Stretching makes sense even on the purely mechanical level of muscle use. Relaxed muscles are stronger and use energy more efficiently. Blood flows more freely to healthy muscles bringing oxygen and nutrients that enable muscles to do their work. Stretching *before* and *after* sports activities enhances performance. Tight muscles are always more easily injured.

Stretching supports the mental game too. The physical sensations of energy and vigor mentally translate into attitude — a can-do confidence that enhances performance. When you are relaxed, balanced and flexible, your state of bodily readiness is also felt as a mental edge.

Top athletes and coaches throughout the world recognize the immediate and long-term benefits of this approach. As Cecil M. Colwin writes in *Swimming into the 21st Century*, "A holistic approach to sports education may permit tomorrow's athletes to tap reserves of power in the human mind and body."[5]

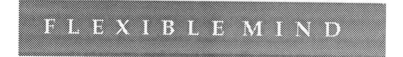

FLEXIBLE MIND

Flexibility as an emotional, mental characteristic has everything to do with reaching beyond limitations. As you practice physical stretches you'll be able to move in ways that may have earlier been out of bounds for you. What would you really like to be able to do? Touch your toes? Do a split? If your inclination is to say, "never in a million years" you may be thinking too inflexibly. To demonstrate the flexible potential of your mind and your body, set yourself a "stretching" challenge.

Sit in the Position of Strength. Your head is positioned directly over your shoulders, your back is straight and your feet are flat on the floor, about shoulder width apart.

Now, inhale as you take a deep Soft Stomach Breath. Slowly exhale as you let your head slowly fall forward. Feel the tightness at the base of the neck, between your shoulders.

When you feel you have had a good stretch, return your head to the upright position.

Do this procedure two more times, and notice how the muscles between your shoulders, at the base of the neck, gradually loosen.

Anyone can stretch, and anyone can realize the benefits from this health-giving process. A mental image may aid your stretching. Try picturing something loose and relaxed or elastic and rubbery, as you relax into the stretch — an old rag doll, a large rubber band. Think positively, give yourself time, relax and do it. In the process you just may let go of some preconceived ideas of what you can and can not do.

MENTAL FLEXIBILITY

A capacity for flexible thinking lies at the heart of discovery. Reflecting on the distinguishing characteristics of high intellectual achievement, science writer James Gleick says: "Children and scientists share an outlook in life. If I do this, what will happen? is both motto of the child at play and the defining refrain of the physical scientist."[6]

The desire to find new ways to solve old problems, is basic to progress, especially in science. A good example of this is the Nobel Prize winning discovery of the structure of the heredity molecule DNA by James Watson and Francis Crick. Watson's own account of this discovery emphasizes the role of creative flexibility in scientific thinking.

Having followed numerous avenues of exploration to figure out the structure of the complex molecule, each ending in fruitless results, Watson tried something new that facilitated one of the greatest scientific discoveries of the 20th century. "The next morning, however, as I took apart a particularly repulsive backbone-centered molecule, I decided that no harm could come from spending a few days building backbone-out models."[7] This shift in his approach to the problem was crucial to unlocking the mystery he eventually solved. Even without understanding the technical details of this shift in viewpoint, we can recognize the importance of an attitude: the willingness to try new ways.

One does not have to look far to find validation of the value of flexibility. It may very well be a fundamental quality of genius. It's a quality that Nobel Prize physicist Richard Feynman, for example, demonstrated to an extraordinary degree. He continuously questioned accepted scientific thinking and left his mark on every area of modern physics.

What was it about this man that so dramatically set him apart from his colleagues? It was Feynman's exceptionally open, questioning mind that is most relevant here. His biographer finds fascinating and amusing evidence of this early on. For example, as captain of his high school math team, Feynman excelled in finding rapid answers to complex problems involving nothing more than standard algebra. Success depended on mental flexibility, on indirectness, solving through subconscious processes, through mental flashes rather than through tedious, conscious, calculations. He felt strongly we must remove rigidity of thought by allowing our mind freedom to wander when trying to solve problems. In this arena, Feynman had no equal and was referred to by his classmates as the "Mad Genius."

Feynman's approach to problem solving was to always question. He felt those who could entertain different theories to explain a single phenomenon had a distinct advantage when in search of new explanations. It has been said of Feynman that he was the most original mind of his time. We have much to learn from his way of thinking.

PARADIGM SHIFTS

Throughout academic and business circles, it is common to hear reference to Thomas S. Kuhn's book, *The Structure of Scientific Revolutions.*[8] When such revolutions occur, we refer to them as "paradigm shifts," changes from one basic way of thinking to another. One such shift occurred when Copernicus concluded our world was not the center of the universe. While his conception of the universe was heretical at the time, Copernicus gradually earned acceptance as his ideas proved to be useful and true. Einstein's theory of relativity brought yet another shift regarding our view of ourselves within the larger scheme of things.

Paradigm shifts represent profound changes in our outlook. They are the fruit of clear, fresh thinking about assumptions which are generally accepted unquestioningly. By encouraging flexibility and alternate ways of thinking, we prepare the way for keener insights into truth and more effective ways of behaving.

Flexibility is a state of readiness, a stance from which you may move in many directions. Clinging to the familiar, the well established, can lead to paralysis or lack of progress. As with rigid, shortened muscles, the ability to move is restricted. Opening up to new possibilities demands a relaxation of preconceptions.

AGING AND MENTAL INFLEXIBILITY

As we grow older, there appears to be a natural inclination to become less flexible, both mentally and physically. This is not a bad thing in itself; in some respects it is necessary for survival and development. Even in our earliest infancy, cells in the body take on special, limited functions in order for the whole body to develop. In our brains, certain neural connections and patterns are reinforced while many others fade away. As we learn our native language we practice reducing the vast variety of impressions and perceptions to manageable order and limits.

We attach names to things and these labels create a simple shorthand for ordering our knowledge. And as we generalize from perceptions to concepts we are able to understand and manage more of our experience in the world.

But in the process of learning and specialization, we risk becoming prisoners of habitual and limiting ways of thinking. The originality with which the child sees the world — the openness and lack of preconception — is often forgotten and obscured by our advancing ability to label and categorize everything we see. This freshness is not lost to us, but it can certainly grow rusty from disuse — unless we value flexibility enough to cultivate it.

SOFT EYES AND HARD EYES REVISITED

One way to practice flexibility is to become aware of the quality of your perception. How observant are you really? Are you quick in sizing up the scene? Do you make snap judgements about what you see? Or do you spend time looking all around taking in the whole picture, and then narrow in on important details?

To gain the truest picture in any situation you need flexibility. You need to see with "hard eyes" and with "soft eyes." In the chapter on Relaxation, we mentioned the martial artist's training in using "hard eyes" and "soft eyes." With hard eyes, your visual focus narrows to concentrate intense awareness on a specific thing. To read the words on this page, for instance, your eyes must narrowly focus on a few small, black marks. With soft eyes, your focus is relaxed and wide; your peripheral vision is enlarged. You can take in a whole roomful of information, but the details may be lost. You would be unable to read this page and take a quick inventory of the room at the same time. They are two different abilities, and we need to be able to do both. Luckily we have this flexibility to shift from narrow, high focus to broad, low focus. That was the point of the exercise in Relaxation.

Let's try the exercise again, but with an additional twist:

Select an object in your immediate environment to focus on. Study it carefully and examine the elements that make it what it is. Notice the shape, color, and anything else that comes to your attention. Focused attention leads to enhanced awareness of detail and structure.

Next, take a few Soft Stomach Breaths and allow your perception to broaden as you relax. Continue your attention to the object, but allow yourself to perceive other things within your 180 degree perceptual span. This requires a relaxed, open attitude.

Now, try alternating back and forth, from the specific object to the general background, from narrow to wide focus. This requires flexibility.

The attitude you are cultivating here is alertness to what is in your field of view, unhampered by preconceptions. It is a critical skill for the martial artist or warrior who must be ready to meet challenges from any direction, but must discriminate between a real threat and a mere distraction or diversion. And it is equally important in mental activity to be completely attentive to what is before us, but alert and open to its meaning and significance. In dealing with people or ideas, prejudgment and misjudgment prevent us from correctly perceiving our situation and our options. Flexibility helps to keep us from shutting down our thinking.

HIGH AND LOW FOCUS THINKING

This ability to shift quickly from narrow to broad visual focus is a built in capacity of human physiology. A parallel flexibility is built into our mental processing as well. As with vision, we are able to think in both highly focused, and broadly diffused ways. We engage in highly focused logical thinking, but we also daydream. Both ways of thinking are important to human effectiveness.

Our capacity for both high and low focus thinking, and our ability to move freely, even playfully, between them is one of the wonderful qualities of our thought. It is, in fact, one of the most mysterious and inimitable capacities of our minds. This interesting observation comes — perhaps not surprisingly — from a leading computer scientist, David Gelernter.[9]

For designers of computers, the ultimate goal is a machine that emulates human thinking. And yet, as most people know, computers are far from capable of thinking as we do. They can perform certain narrow, highly focused tasks like mathematical computation much faster than we can. But most of the mental feats we perform without a second thought — for example, instantly connecting the momentary sound of a voice we haven't heard for years with a person we haven't even thought of for a long time — are way beyond any computer. This is why computer scientists and theorists of artificial intelligence have had to go back to basics to learn more about how we think.

That's what led Professor Gelernter to his observations about high and low focus thinking. It's a step toward analyzing the elusive ways the human brain can make lightning leaps of insight, creativity, and imagination. High focus thought is intensely narrowed, penetrating in its logical analysis. Low focus thinking brings in emotions, associations, sensations, memories — the very human element which is missing from machines. Like soft eyes, it gives us instant access to an immense range of information and stimuli outside the tunnel vision of logic. This continuous range of focus and the capability to adjust it is what makes our brains so much richer, more unpredictable, and more powerful than computers.

Fortunately we don't have to be able to analyze our brains in order to use them, but we do have to use them to the fullest in order to be all we are capable of. And it's when we are freely using our full mental capacity that we truly feel we are in the zone. Many of us, however, neglect and undervalue our low focus thinking. Intuition, fantasy and daydreaming have gotten a bad rap in our fast-paced culture. This is a shame since low focus thinking is the wellspring of creativity.

THE IMPORTANCE OF YOUR IMAGINATION

All of us have a lot more brain power than we'll ever use. So it's important to know that even people who are considered the brainiest among us recognize that their best thinking involves not just high focus logic, but the entire spectrum of thought, especially imagination. Indeed, it's this openness to the whole range of thinking that really gives us access to our own great mental capacity.

Albert Einstein is frequently mentioned as an example of a highly rational thinker who relied heavily on his imagination in arriving at his most significant insights. He himself often spoke of the absolutely crucial role of this kind of thinking in his work. "When I examine myself and my methods of thought," he said, "I come to the conclusion that the gift of fantasy has meant more to me than my talent for absorbing positive knowledge."[10]

EINSTEIN DID IT, SO CAN YOU

So how do we get our imaginations going? How do we limber up those seemingly rigid thought patterns and get out of the old mental ruts? Many of us believe that imaginative freedom is something we outgrow, or leave behind us like a much-loved, worn out toy.

You can rest assured that no matter how rusty it may be, your imagination is still in good working order. The main thing is just to let yourself use it.

We can make it easier for ourselves by following Einstein's example: first, relax. As we noted in the chapter on Relaxation, he deliberately sought out environments and activities like sailing and playing music which provided a change of pace. Relaxation was not an escape from unsolved problems; it was an integral part of the process of solving them.

STIMULATING YOUR IMAGINATION

Of course there are many ways to engage and activate your imagination. It's not our purpose to explore all of them here. We'll keep it simple by recalling that the ability to form mental images is a key ingredient of creative thought. This is true in the arts as well as sciences, and also offers a powerful source of creativity in your everyday life. Your ability to imagine new possibilities shapes your ever-changing conception of the options available to you, of what you might become.

Here's a simple exercise you can use to activate your ability to form images. If it seems too simple-minded you can easily come up with more sophisticated variants. But as I said before, the main thing is to jump-start your imagination.

As in previous exercises, you will benefit from relaxation which reduces barriers to imaging. Assume the Position of Comfort and do a few deep Soft Stomach Breaths. If someone can read the following to you, it will be useful. If not, just read on:

What? *— Imagine you are some specific thing. It doesn't matter what it is. Get a clear picture before you move on.*

Where? *— Where is it? Be sure you picture it in relation to a specific environment.*

Why? *— Why is it there? There can be many reasons. Select one that makes sense to you.*

When? *— When is it? What century, year, month, day, time of day?*

Feelings? *— How does it feel, or does it not have feelings? In either case, what is it like to feel or not feel?*

Movement? *— Is it going anywhere or will it always be where it is?*

The point of this exercise is to demonstrate imagination is an active process, under your control. You can activate your imagination at any time. Suppose you want to solve a problem, write a poem or a song, invent or do something innovative. Or suppose you want to play out a scenario for some course of action you might pursue.

You don't need a computer program. You've got something better already right there between your ears. It's the inherent flexibility of your mind. Use it to change your perspective, to expand your possibilities, to discover creative alternatives through active orchestration of your imagination, whenever you want.

FOCUS

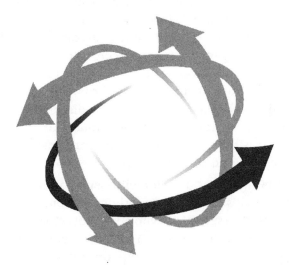

FOCUS

If you ask people, as I have, what they think of when they hear the phrase *In the Zone,* most answer that it has to do with being completely focused on what you are doing. You are concentrating. You are so "in to" it that your mind and body are acting in total unity. You've blocked out everything else. In fact, an attitude of complete focus and concentration seems to be virtually synonymous with being in the zone.

Where do we see people who are really focused? Sports comes quickly to mind, whether you're an active or an armchair athlete. When you see great athletic accomplishments you know you're seeing moments of total concentration of mind and body. Think of a pass receiver in football reaching for the ball with every fiber of his being, knowing he is about to be hit by a 200 pound safety. Think of the Olympic discus thrower who must combine intricate steps, timing, muscular movements, breath and spirit in one whirling, explosive moment which will determine the world championship.

Sports are a great arena for witnessing focused action. In fact, I think that's one of the underlying reasons for the great appeal of sports to spectators who might not actually engage in a particular sport themselves. You may never hurl yourself headlong down an icy slope in competitive downhill skiing, or push your body to the limits day after day in bicycling's Tour de France, or stand up to a pitcher throwing a scorching 98 mile an hour fastball. But you can sense the effort of concentration required to perform those feats.

Of course sports isn't the only arena where we see and appreciate focused action. We gauge actors' performances by the degree to which they immerse themselves in their parts and identify with their roles. Musicians play their best when they become one with the music. Regardless of the kind of music they play, we recognize and respond to their total concentration in their performance.

IT'S EXHILARATING AND WE ALL KNOW IT

I don't mean to suggest that focus is something we see only in top performers and highly trained specialists. On the contrary, I think we recognize and respond to it intuitively, because it is something we are all familiar with in our own experience. The feeling of being totally concentrated on something is actually one of the most exhilarating and rewarding feelings we can experience, and I think it's a feeling that many people crave without being quite aware of it.

Think about times when you have been totally involved in what you were doing and thinking, pretty much to the exclusion of any other thought. How about a time when you have been in love, or in ecstasy or, at the other extreme, in danger, in pain, in agony, in despair. These are moments, like many in childhood, where you are completely immersed in the action and feeling of the moment, where there is no separation and distinction between who you are and what you experience.

BUT CAN WE DO IT WHENEVER WE WANT?

However, these are extreme situations, which are not quite what we mean by focus — because they tend to be situations in which we are not in control. What we mean by focus also includes the critical element of being in charge, in command. We want the intensity and the power of focused thought and action—and we want to control that intensity and power, to use it at will.

The power to focus, to bring ourselves entirely into our situation or task at any given moment, is what distinguishes a high level from an erratic, unreliable performance. Many of us use this power in particular, highly specialized fields of activity. Like the athlete or performer, the surgeon or artist must concentrate all their precise manual skills and trained judgement in real time action. Any activity where success or failure depends on the extent to which you are "all there" requires the ability to focus.

On the job, the manager whose mind wanders will miss critical moments of awareness and decision. The salesperson who can't concentrate with full attention on the customer in the moment of trying to make a sale is unlikely to succeed. At home, the parent who can't, in the presence of his child, bring his complete attention to being there for that child, is shortchanging his child and himself. And in any personal relationship, if we can't truly focus on the other person and the relationship between us, that relationship will sooner or later become an empty shell and a charade.

So it's essential to be able to focus when you want to focus, to concentrate when you need to. That's the critical power that enables you to perform your best at will, so that when you want and need to be, you can be — in the zone.

IT'S A SKILL YOU'VE BEEN BUILDING

You can. In fact the relaxation, balance, and flexibility skills and habits you've been practicing will take you a long way towards cultivating the power of concentration. At first glance, relaxation might seem completely opposed to focus. But remember the saying, "Relaxation equals the peak of efficiency." Physically, we operate most efficiently when we have no friction or hindrance of any kind. Similarly, mental concentration is at its peak when the mind is clear of all tensions and obstacles.

Focus also relies on balance — on using the power of the center to align forces and produce a unified powerful action. At the physical level, focus of motion is achieved through coordination of breathing and full body movement from our center of gravity. Mentally, focus requires the marshalling of resources, making choices and decisions that advance our central purpose.

As we saw in the chapter on flexibility, concentration is at the high end of a continuous range of thought, the region of penetrating and purposeful thinking. Flexibility allows us to shift easily and quickly from generalized awareness to sharply defined attention. Think of a magnifying glass which gathers light and directs it in concentrated beam to one precise spot. You can set a fire with this concentrated energy. Your thoughts and actions can achieve the same power of focus.

FOCUSED BODY

FOCUSING STRENGTH IN ACTION

When movement, breath control, and full body posture are unified in a single focused act, then physical power is maximized. In the martial arts there is a characteristic "yell" commonly referred to as *ki-ai*. It is typically used at the moment of delivering a punch or kick, for greater power, coordination and protection against injury.

When you **Exhale Into The Exertion**, into a **Hard Stomach Breath** as is done in a *ki-ai*, you are contracting your abdominal muscles. This muscular contraction strengthens connections between the upper and lower halves of your body. Thus, your body becomes a single unit and physical power is focused through your center.

In this chapter you'll be practicing many such focusing exercises and increasing your ability to concentrate, — concentrate force and concentrate attention. The exercises apply to a wide variety of physical and mental activities. You will quickly see just how to use these skills in your own personal life. Begin by trying this basic exercise.

HARD STOMACH BREATHING

In the sitting position, place your hands flat on your thighs. Take a deep Soft Stomach Breath. Now exhale fully as you press down on your thighs. Notice how your abdominal muscles gradually tighten as you Exhale Into The Exertion and press downward. You have coordinated your breathing with the body movement of pressing downward.

Contrast this with the following experience:

*Place your hands on your thighs. Take a deep Soft Stomach Breath and **hold your breath** as you press down on your thighs. Notice the pressure that builds up just below your rib cage and above your belt line.*

Do you notice a difference between these two exercises? People typically hold their breath during times of exertion, even though it is far more effective and safer to Exhale Into The Exertion. When you take a Soft Stomach Breath, stomach muscles loosen and spread out, becoming more diffuse. This relaxes your stomach area making it soft and vulnerable. In sports for example, a blow to that soft area would be particularly disabling. When you are struck in your "hardened" stomach, your tightened muscles protect you because they form a sheath of contracted muscle tissue.

THIS KIND OF PROTECTION MONEY CAN'T BUY

You may have noticed the common tendency of employers to buy "back" support belts (which are really "abdominal" support belts) for employees who lift on the job. Despite evidence these belts do not help the wearer lift more weight, and are ineffective in preventing back injuries without training in correct body mechanics and lifting techniques, employers continue to buy these belts by the thousands.

It makes more sense to learn how to use your body correctly. When you Exhale Into The Exertion, abdominal muscles contract, providing built in abdominal support for the low back. You become stronger and safer as you develop habits of correct breathing.

Another advantage of Hard Stomach Breathing is that as you exhale, air pressure within your body is reduced. Reduced internal pressure, along with tightened abdominal muscles, provides protection against a hiatal hernia (a condition in which a portion of the stomach pushes through the diaphragm into the chest cavity).

When you integrate Soft and Hard Stomach breathing with physical activity, you engage in "Power Breathing."[1] It is a powerful breathing technique, useful throughout your work day, home life and during sports.

THE POWER BREATHING KATA

In the chapter on balance, we introduced the Position of Strength Kata to help you practice basic movements that maintain your balance as your position shifts. In traditional martial arts training, as we said, katas are sequences of basic body postures and movements, practiced so that they can be performed fluidly and seamlessly without conscious thought. Now I would like to extend this Position of Strength Kata with additional movements that will train you to Exhale Into The Exertion as you move.

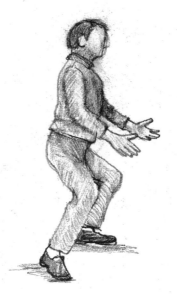

Rising From A Crouch

The following series of specific, correct movements will teach you to lift, bend, push and pull in a safe, effective manner. Practice the movements slowly and deliberately, as if you are performing before an audience. Notice your feelings of concentration, both mental and physical, as you practice these sequences.

First, check for muscle tension, and limber up with stretches if necessary. Relax your mind and body with Soft Stomach Breaths. Find your center of gravity with a Hard Stomach Breath. Then begin:

RISING FROM A CROUCH

Take a Soft Stomach Breath as you bend your knees and lower yourself to a moderate crouch position.

*Slowly exhale into a Hard Stomach Breath as you push yourself up to the fully vertical position. You are **Exhaling Into The Exertion**.*

*Imagine you have a heavy barbell on your shoulders while performing this exercise. Remember to **keep your chest slightly forward** at all times to maintain that important low back curve.*

PUSHING

Practice Power Breathing in the Position of Strength as you imagine yourself pushing something at each side of your body.

Widen your stance to increase stability. Your chest is slightly forward and knees are slightly bent.

Inhale with a Soft Stomach Breath and slowly exhale into a Hard Stomach Breath as you imagine yourself pushing against pillars on both sides of you. Imagine you are Samson pushing against the pillars of the temple. Why not? Have a little fun.

Now, imagine pushing a refrigerator in front of you. Exhale Into The Exertion as you push, and remember always to maintain a widened stance and a relaxed, balanced, full body attitude.

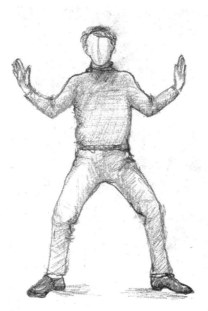

Pushing

PULLING

Enter the Position of Strength and imagine you are engaged in a tug of war.

Drop one foot back to widen your stance. This gives you balance and power.

Keep your chest slightly forward as you pull and Exhale Into The Exertion.

To increase pulling power, bend your knees and lower your center of gravity. Use the technique of Sumo Wrestlers.

LIFTING

Practice the Position of Strength and Power Breathing while lifting something from the floor. Most people bend at the

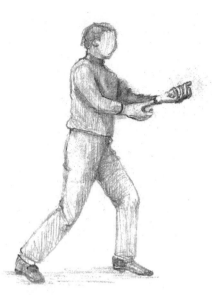

Pulling

waist and lift with their hands and arms. When you bend at the waist into a rounded back position with legs straight, you are in the Position of Weakness. This is hazardous and not an effective way to lift anything. Use the Position of Strength and Power Breathing as you lift.

Imagine you are a weight lifter, lifting a heavy barbell from the floor. Take a Soft Stomach Breath, bend at the knees with chest slightly forward, then Exhale Into The Exertion as you lift and rise to a standing position.

How many times do you bend over in the Position of Weakness to pick up something, when you could be using the Position of Strength? Practice makes perfect. Soon you will be lifting correctly as a matter of habit.

POWER BREATHING IN SPORTS

Regular practice of the Position of Strength (balanced posture) coordinated with Exhaling Into The Exertion (Power

Breathing) will help you to form beneficial habits of correct, full body movements. This self-training will prove useful in all your physical activities. If you want to improve your golf swing, your tennis game, batting average or your bowling score, you will always do better when you use Power Breathing and the Position of Strength.

Athletes and coaches often gain valuable insights that improve their performance by watching skilled specialists in other sports. You can use this mental cross-training too. For example, the chances are that you've never tried fencing, and don't intend to. But if you take a look at fencing technique, you can see a very pure example of the effective use of Power Breathing.

The lunge is one of the fundamental moves in fencing. In simple terms, it is a long step forward with the leading foot as the fencer attempts to reach an opponent with the point of the sword. It is by far the most rapid attack a fencer can make. When a lunge is performed, it is common to hear the fencer make a *ki-ai*-like sound which is, once again, the coordination of breathing, full body movement, and mental concentration.

"THE GRUNT"

Anyone who follows tennis knows of Jimmy Connors and how he often makes a ki-ai like sound as his racket meets the ball. I don't happen to know how and why Connors began this practice, but it's clear that when you serve or return a tennis ball, coordination, timing, power, and accuracy are increased as you Exhale Into The Exertion at the moment of impact.

As other tennis stars picked up this technique, it aroused a lot of notice, not all of it favorable. In August of 1992, USA Today reported "Grunts gone, Seles loses in silence." Monica Seles was the number one woman professional in the world of tennis, winner of six grand slam titles and had gained a certain reputation for her so-called "grunting." Because of media attention and complaints from other players, Seles cut back on her grunting and subsequently lost three consecutive finals. In fact, she lost to a player she had previously beaten ten consecutive times.

Seles had learned the breathing techniques behind the grunt from Sports Psychologist James Loehr, and claims it boosts her intensity and aggressiveness during competition. In defense of Seles, tennis great Chris Evert said, "You need to grunt, and most players do." Similarly, Brett Newman, ranked in the top five in the nation in table tennis, told me "the breathing technique I use, namely Power Breathing, helped me to develop an extremely powerful smash and forehand loop in Table Tennis."

During the 1992 Summer Olympics in Barcelona, sportscasters amused by the "screaming" observed during various competitive events, presented a mini-special on "Olympic Screamers". Power Breathing was observable in the Hammer Throw, Shot Put, Weight Lifting and many other events. "We've got to scream to produce," one Olympian joked. Winning athletes take advantage of any competitive edge.

POWER BREATHING AND GOLF

Ask the average golfer how he or she breathes during a golf swing. The usual response I get to that question is, "I have never thought about it. I guess I don't know."

Imagine you are swinging a golf club. What are your options? Of course, you won't hold your breath. Among other things, holding your breath produces physical tension, the ubiquitous enemy of most golfers. And, you won't inhale as you swing the club forward to hit the ball, because this feels unnatural and reduces power and coordination. There is another option: Inhale comfortably on the backswing and Exhale Into The Exertion comfortably as you swing the club forward and connect with the ball.

Biomechanical computer analysis has proven that the effectiveness of a golf swing depends on coordination of full body movements around your center of gravity. That's precisely what Power Breathing does. Coordinating correct breathing technique with correct body mechanics increases your accuracy and strength and improves your game, because you function more directly from your center.

Incidentally, if you are a golfer, use Soft Stomach Breathing while putting. Focus on relaxed, rhythmic breathing before and during putting and you will increase accuracy. A relaxed, full body attitude is the name of the game.

FROM ARCHERY TO HORSE SHOES

Archery is one sport in which there is a long tradition of training to acquire both physical and mental discipline, particularly in the Orient. Kenneth Kushner describes this training in his book *One Arrow, One Life*.[2] Here is his careful explanation of the role of Power Breathing in the archer's release of the arrow.

The force of the breath necessary to make a loud ki-ai emphasizes the force of breath necessary for a proper release. . . . At the point of release there should be a sense of unity between one's breathing, posture and concentration.

Kushner, like Sally Swift whose techniques of Centered Riding we mentioned in the chapters on Relaxation and Balance, began the study of a sport for personal reasons. Kushner sought to improve poor posture through training in archery which requires good posture. Sally Swift was motivated by a back problem involving an abnormal curvature of the spine. By studying how the mind can control deep inner muscles, and how posture, body balance, center of gravity, relaxation and breathing interrelate, both achieved excellence of athletic technique along with improved health.

There is an ancient Samurai saying, "Mastery of an Art is revealed in your every action." Mastery of breathing techniques has application in many aspects of your daily activities. Since you are breathing throughout your day anyway, why not do it correctly and use it to your advantage.

In the course of years of giving seminars in corporations around the country, I've encountered many people who have been excited by making this connection. One participant in a training program in Tennessee, a man who had been a top contender in state level bowling competition for several years told me, "I have been bowling for years and have never considered how my breathing could have anything to do with proper bowling technique." Another individual, an executive with a national railroad was delighted to find that "Power Breathing also works in horse shoes."

POWER BREATHING IN EVERYDAY ACTIVITIES

Power Breathing is applicable during all body movements that require you to exert yourself. Every time you lift, push, pull, throw, kick, hit, etc., you should remind yourself to focus your energy by Exhaling Into The Exertion while in the Position

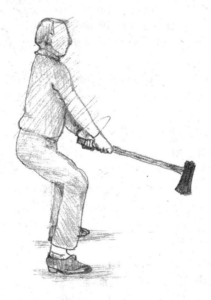

Chopping Wood

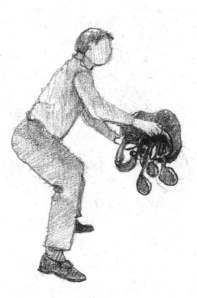

Lifting Golf Clubs

of Strength. You will experience greater power, control over your body movements and increased self-protection. This advice holds for all manner of sports as well as everyday routine activities.

LIFTING A CHAIR

Stand behind a chair. As you reach for the chair, keep your chest slightly forward, and Exhale Into The Exertion as you lift the chair. Focus on Power Breathing while lifting.

As you set the chair down, be sure to keep your chest slightly forward and Exhale Into The Exertion. It is easy to forget this when we set things down, but those are times of exertion too.

EVEN WHILE LYING DOWN

You are lying on the floor watching television. You want to use this time productively and also want to exercise abdominal muscles. Enter The Position of Comfort. Take a deep Soft Stomach Breath and slowly exhale. Continue to exhale as you progress to a Hard Stomach Breath. Continue exhaling until your stomach muscles are fully contracted and your low back is flat against the floor. You have Exhaled Into The Exertion and have put abdominal muscles to work. You are practicing Power Breathing and are giving abdominal muscles a slight workout. If you count your exhalations during this exercise, you are practicing concentration skills as well; not an easy task while watching television.

Think of how Power Breathing could be of benefit in the following activities:

Chopping wood,

Shoveling snow,

Lifting a baby out of a crib,

Pushing a refrigerator,

Lifting golf clubs from the trunk of your car.

You can easily add to this list. Remember, you are exploring how to function from your center. Power Breathing, through exhalation and tightened stomach muscles, coordinates your body movements around your center of gravity. This makes you physically more powerful and provides important support for your spine at the belt line.

FOCUSED MIND

Even more important is the mental concentration that comes with the unification of all your capacities into a singular concerted action. When you are relaxed, balanced, flexible and focused, your muscles, respiration, oxygen consumption, heart rate, blood flow, neural messages, emotions and thoughts all work in concert. You are in the zone. It's not too hard to see the value of this unity — in any activity, at any level of skill.

FEEL YOUR PULSE

Here is quick exercise that will give you the pleasure of experiencing mental and physical focus in a very simple way:

Sit in the Position of Strength, which means your chest is slightly forward and you have a nice inward curve in your lower back. Put your hands together in your lap so that your fingers are interlocked and your index fingers are touching at the ends.

Inhale with a Soft Stomach Breath and hold it briefly. Slowly exhale, and as you do so, use your ability to relax to eliminate tension. Concentrate on the focal point between your index fingers. Feel your pulse there.

You may have difficulty feeling the pulse at first, so take another deep Soft Stomach Breath and slowly exhale. Close your eyes if you feel it helps you to concentrate on that point. As your pulse comes into focus, you are becoming increasingly centered. Through breathing, mental concentration and your physical sensations, you are becoming aware of your body as an integrated, single unit. This is a good example of Focused Action.

As you probably know, this exercise is similar to many meditative practices that are common to cultures all over the world. It is the basis of many spiritual and mental disciplines such as Yoga (which actually comes from the ancient Sanskrit word for *yoke* or *union* of mind and body) and Zen (the core of which is concentration of mind and body in one-pointed action) as well as prayer and meditation in Western spirituality. But this and similar exercises do not have particular religious connotations, or involve any set of beliefs. People in all times and cultures have used them because they have been proven to be effective for unifying mind and body.

TOTAL FOCUS

Before we go further we should mention a familiar, but seemingly paradoxical fact about concentration. Trying to concentrate can be like trying to relax: worrying about whether or not you're doing it right can get in the way of actually doing it. One must simply be focused, which means, pay full attention to what you are doing in that moment.

PITCHING PENNIES

Here's a variant on an old pastime that will help you to experience the difference between merely thinking about being focused and actually developing the feeling of focus.

Gather a handful of pennies. Place a receptacle on the floor. (An empty tin can or plastic food storage container is a handy size.) Stand or sit in the Position of Strength a moderately challenging distance away.

Relax and take regular, rhythmic breaths. Focus exclusively on the can and release the pennies as you exhale. Don't worry about missing. And don't concentrate on concentrating, but get into the rhythm and "flow" of it all. Continue as long as you like.

How did it go? When you began, did your attempts to become focused get in the way? Was there a point at which your concentration really jelled, a point at which you became totally absorbed in the game? Did your aim improve as a consequence?

LETTING GO TO GET IN FOCUS

Many people experience focus as a kind of letting go of self. The "I" as doer becomes absorbed in the doing. Novelists have spoken of this sensation in the creative process. Writing can become so intensely focused that the characters seemingly take over and tell their own stories. The words simply flow and can be channeled through the fingertips and onto the page. That's concentration!

This total absorption, when the self is merged with the action it is performing, is not unique to writing. It's an integral part of any kind of intense concentration. In moments of pure focus nothing is wasted on doubt, self-criticism and self-consciousness. Operation is at peak efficiency, more can be achieved with less. There's an ease of effort and an absence of tension. Only those faculties that need to be operating are consuming energy.

YOU CAN ACTUALLY SEE THIS IN A BRAIN SCAN

Do you need to see this to believe it? With the new technology of Positron Emission Tomography (PET Scanning) we can actually see comparative pictures of mental efficiency. A PET Scan is a graphic picture of a brain's energy consumption. On the PET Scan, red coloration shows the highest degree of energy consumption, followed by orange, yellow, green and down the rainbow spectrum. The more complex the task, the more energy is consumed by the brain.

Pet Scans that compare novice performers with skilled performers of the same task show marked difference in energy consumption. Novices have redder, hotter scans. They consume more energy and involve many more brain areas in carrying out the task. Skilled performers on the other hand show cooler, less active scans. Energy consumption is minimized. Greater skill requires less energy, leads to greater focus and requires less overall brain activity.

So we come to the question of skill and its relationship to focus. Nothing will aid your concentration better than practice, practice, practice of your craft or sport or discipline. You can't fake a good performance. If your skill in a particular activity is undeveloped, doubt may creep in and ruin your focus. But on the other hand, your ability to focus will make or break your performance at even a high degree of skill. So it's useful to find practical ways to increase your concentration, no matter how advanced your mastery of a discipline.

Even if you've never before deliberately tried to sharpen your concentration, you are already well on your way if you've been able to improve your ability to be relaxed, balanced, and flexible. As we said early in this chapter, concentration is a skill that not only can be learned, but is built on these three other core skills of relaxation, balance and flexibility. In fact they provide an indispensable foundation for the development of focusing skills. They make it possible to lessen self-consciousness, suspend judgement, become completely absorbed in the activity, and enjoy yourself in the process.

HOW YOUR BRAIN BLOCKS OUT DISTRACTIONS

Human beings have very acute senses. At any moment our eyes, ears, nose, skin are exposed to myriad stimuli. Think of all the distractions you could be subject to if you chose to. You have the capacity to focus on any particular square inch of your skin at will. What would happen if every nerve ending in your foot screamed for attention, alerting you to the fact that it was resting on the floor? Luckily we can forget about how the bottoms of our feet feel and only have to think about them when we decide we need to. We have as much capacity to block out stimulation as we do to attend to it.

Concentration is often a function of how well we block out distractions. Built into our nervous system is a special ability to do just this: block out unimportant sensations. Our nerve cells secrete a specific neurotransmitter called GABA (gamma amino butyric acid) that makes the nervous system less sensitive to stimuli. We activate the release of GABA when we immerse ourselves in an activity. Then GABA allows us to maintain our focus by desensitizing us to our surroundings.[3] That's why time flies when you're having fun — or doing anything else absorbing. GABA blocks out distraction. Focus is not an alien state. We're really set up to focus, we just need to practice it.

Release of GABA is a learned response. As children we have short, easily distracted attention spans. As we mature, we are able to focus more readily on the tasks necessary for learning and working. The ability to secrete GABA increases with practice as you actively learn how to focus.

Create occasions to practice concentration. Establish a quiet time and find a stress-free environment. Practice focusing activities. Practice focus in conjunction with a skill you are learning, or try some of the focusing activities in this book. Many people find contemplation a wonderful way to refresh themselves and sustain attention. Prayer and meditation are time honored practices that have perennially nourished the human spirit.

LIVING IN THE ZONE

When you are focused, you "know" what is required and "do" what it takes to get it done. When you are hungry, you search for food, and satisfy your needs. You are goal directed. You can do what is necessary without fuss, distraction, and bungling. Your attention is on what you are doing. You are integrated mentally, physically, and emotionally — focused in the moment.

Does this seem like too far-fetched and unrealistic a goal? It isn't. It's the way we all function best, the way we were born to be, the way we can most enjoy our life, whatever its unique circumstances. The purpose of this book is no more and no less than to show you that. The power to be in the zone whenever and wherever we choose is something we all possess. Use it.

LIVING IN THE ZONE

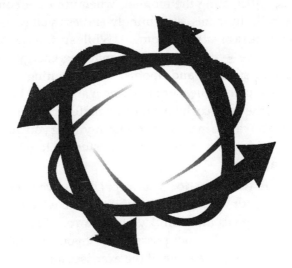

LIVING IN THE ZONE

It's the bottom of the ninth — score is tied, three balls and two strikes — the possibility of a hit, even a home run. "Just me and the Pitcher!" I'm in the zone.

Living in the zone is your opportunity to live life to the fullest, moment by moment, to take each step along your way with clear vision, purpose, intense commitment. When in the zone, you are fully focused on what you are doing. It's your total readiness, anticipating the moment when your bat connects with the ball. In tennis, a seemingly endless volley, as each return stretches a breathless moment. While surfing, in the curl of a great wave — captured within spiraling energy — then released into sunlight and another wave waiting. In rifle marksmanship, the squeeze of the trigger and a neat bulls eye. In billiards, the three cushion bank and perfect position for the next shot. You can be in the zone doing anything you do. It can be while playing your favorite sport, listening to your mate, watching a sunset.

You are what you do. Your capacity to live completely results from your willingness and ability to do what it takes to achieve your goals and fulfill your dreams. The tools are simple, and already in your possession. If you have taken the opportunity to practice some of the exercises and ideas in the previous sections of this book, you will hopefully have gotten a feel for the way relaxation, balance, flexibility and focus can be naturally attained and used in your life.

A FULL BODY ATTITUDE

You have learned the Position of Strength and how chest forward, knees bent, with arms close to your body provide a full body posture, useful in all action situations. You know to **move from the pelvis first**. Quickness of body movements, power and accuracy are determined, by your ability to move from your center. Consider the following:

FULL BODY MOVEMENTS IN TENNIS

As the ball comes to you, move from the pelvis first. This means moving your total body as a single unit. When body movements originate from your center, you automatically move your upper body in concert with your lower body. You arrive at the spot where you return the ball with perfect posture. Your carriage is erect, rather than twisted and bent forward. Your feet are directly under your center of gravity, just as your head is directly above it. You make your return with full power, speed and accuracy.

RELAXED, FULL BODY ATTITUDE

Full body movements, driven by a full body attitude, are essential to peak performances. These same **full body movements must be relaxed**, fluent, and delivered with ease. We have discussed relaxed breathing and how the physical state of relaxation is facilitated by correct breathing.

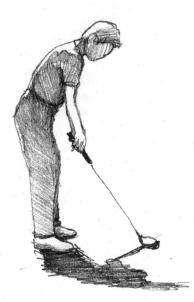

RELAXED GOLFER

You are in the Position of Strength and know your swing must be relaxed and fully coordinated around your center of gravity; full body movements must be integrated with your breathing. Relax your body with a few deep Soft Stomach Breaths. Stand up to the ball — slowly inhale during the back swing — Exhale Into The Exertion as you complete your forward swing.

CONCENTRATED FULL BODY MOVEMENTS

We push cars stuck in snow, move furniture, lift young children, hit home runs. In each situation, we have ourselves and the object of our attention. Consider the following:

HITTING A BASEBALL

You are relaxed in the Position of Strength. As the ball approaches, you begin your relaxed swing. Exhale Into The Exertion as your bat and the ball meet. You are relaxed, balanced, flexible, focused and engaged in full body movement.

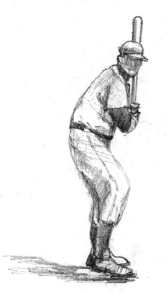

CHOPPING WOOD

*Stand in the Position of Strength. With the axe positioned directly in front of you, slowly raise the axe to the upright position. Your focus is the middle of the log to be split. **Exhale Into The Exertion** as you bring the axe into contact with the log. Let the axe, the forces of gravity, and your coordinated full body movements do the work.*

ACTIVITIES OF DAILY LIVING

Analyze your physical movements on a typical day. One third of the time you are asleep. That is a full body posture, horizontal to the pull of gravity on your body. What about the remaining two thirds of your time? Most of us are sitting or standing.

IN THE ZONE WHILE SITTING

Consider the following:

Your hands are on the keyboard and you are typing a letter. Mentally you are focused on words as they appear on the screen. Physically, your body is positioned correctly. Your chest is forward, which also facilitates good low back posture. Your hands are parallel to the keyboard, eliminating unnecessary strain in your wrists and shoulders. Emotionally, you are relaxed.

As the day wears on, tedium sets in, physical tensions mount, and you gradually slump into your chair.

Stop! Resume good posture. Push your chest forward and straighten your back. Relax with a few deep Soft Stomach Breaths. Once again, you are in the zone where you do your best work.

IN THE ZONE WHILE STANDING

If you are not lying down or sitting, most likely you are in a vertical position where it is easy to slump into awkward postures. Consider the following:

You are a bank teller. You stand much of your working day. As the day wears on, tension accumulates and you feel increasingly uncomfortable. Now is the time to push your chest forward, bend your knees slightly and take a few deep Soft Stomach Breaths. Relax and center yourself. Once again, you are in the zone.

YOUR FAVORITE PHYSICAL ACTIVITY

Among the many things you like to do, surely one activity must stand out as your favorite. Tennis, golf, weight lifting, gardening, walking, running, hiking, bowling. The list of possibilities is virtually endless.

> What is your favorite physical activity?
>
> Do you use the Position of Strength during this activity?
>
> Are you relaxed?
>
> Do you use Soft Stomach Breathing?
>
> Do you ExhaleInto The Exertion?
>
> Do you feel well coordinated?
>
> Are you flexible?
>
> Are you using full body movements?

Remember, no matter what you are doing, you will do it better when you are relaxed, balanced, flexible and focused.

MIND AND BODY BECOME ONE

When you are in that sweet spot and at the top of your game, when you are at your best, you are in the zone where mind and body function as one. Your mind is focused on what you are doing. Your full body movements are spontaneous and effortless. Soccer star Pelé says it well, "I do nothing; I simply let the body move."[1]

But this is not always easy to do. There are so many things to distract us. The history of great sports moments is replete with situations where highly trained, skilled athletes were challenged during moments of intense competition by other factors. A death in the family, physical problems, lack of adequate sleep, disagreement with a coach, pressures from the media, are among the possible disruptions of total concentration. Despite these obstacles, great athletes deliver great performances on a highly reliable basis, because they remain relaxed, balanced, flexible and focused while performing the task at hand. In sports, this is essential. In our ongoing lives this is a great possibility!

As a Clinical and Sport Psychologist, I have learned over the years, that people seek psychological help for one basic reason, *They don't feel the way they want to feel.* Additionally, they don't have a good grasp of where these feelings are coming from. There is a fundamental lack of connection between the mind and the body. An individual might say, "I am unhappy" when in fact, he is "angry." The first challenge then, is to develop the ability to correctly identify feelings. The remaining challenge is to find out where the feelings come from.

Integrate mind and body experiences through the following focusing technique: This exercise requires concentration and a quiet place. If you have someone read it to you, it will be more effective.

FOCUS ON YOUR FEELINGS

Step One: Close your eyes and take a deep Soft Stomach Breath. Pay attention to your breathing as you inhale and exhale. Do two more Soft Stomach Breaths as you prepare yourself for step two.

Step Two: Pay attention to your body and ask yourself the question, **"How do I feel right now?"** Just feel the answer in your body. Don't analyze it. Just be aware of it.

Step Three: Locate specific parts of your body

where your feelings come from. It might be your heart rate, something in your stomach, in your chest, your arms, neck, your back.

Step Four: From your many feelings, select one and focus on it. Describe it. Say to yourself, **"I feel . . ."** and then complete the sentence.

Step Five: Alternate, back and forth, between the word (i.e., your mental conception) and the feeling (i.e., your physical experience) — the word and the feeling — the word and the feeling. Like an echo between your mind and your body. Notice how you gradually refine the word and the feeling — and they gradually become one. The word perfectly matches the feeling.

Use this mind/body focusing technique to identify your true feelings. Another element of this process of self-awareness is to further explore "where" your feelings might be coming from. This brings us to the challenge of measuring how you feel about a variety of possible personal concerns.

On a scale from 0 to 10, **indicate how comfortable you are with your life today**. 0 means you are totally comfortable and don't feel any tension in your life. 10 means you are very uncomfortable about that item. Choose the number that best relates your level of concern.

$$0 - 1 - 2 - 3 - 4 - 5 - 6 - 7 - 8 - 9 - 10$$

unconcerned   moderately concerned   very concerned

To explore your rating above in greater detail, consider the following 12 broad areas of possible personal concern. Once again, use your feelings as the basic guide for how concerned you really are. Your "gut level" reactions are of great value as

RATE EACH GENERAL AREA OF PERSONAL CONCERN:

Indicate to what degree each general area is a concern of yours today. Use your feelings as your guide. Listen to your feelings, they don't lie!

More Time For Myself   0-1-2-3-4-5-6-7-8-9-10
I am concerned about having more time and space to do my own thing.

Self-Defeating Behaviors   0-1-2-3-4-5-6-7-8-9-10
I am concerned about activities I am involved in that hurt me.

Sexual Difficulties   0-1-2-3-4-5-6-7-8-9-10
I am concerned about problems involving sex.

Financial Problems   0-1-2-3-4-5-6-7-8-9-10
I am concerned about money problems.

Relationship Problems   0-1-2-3-4-5-6-7-8-9-10
I am concerned about my relations with others.

Emotional Problems   0-1-2-3-4-5-6-7-8-9-10
I am concerned about problems I am having expressing or controlling my feelings.

Continuing Health Problems   0-1-2-3-4-5-6-7-8-9-10
I am concerned about physical problems I need to pay attention to.

Difficulty Making Decisions   0-1-2-3-4-5-6-7-8-9-10
I am concerned about my ability to make decisions.

Family Problems   0-1-2-3-4-5-6-7-8-9-10
I am concerned about problems I am having with family members.

Eating Habits   0-1-2-3-4-5-6-7-8-9-10
I am concerned about my eating and drinking habits.

Exercise   0-1-2-3-4-5-6-7-8-9-10
I am concerned about the adequacy of my physical exercise.

The Meaning Of Life   0-1-2-3-4-5-6-7-8-9-10
I am concerned I am not getting what I want out of life.

You just made a brief review of possible personal concerns, gauging your own feelings in each area. You discovered, perhaps, certain concerns you weren't fully aware of. Even though you may have been involved in reading this book, outside concerns were in your consciousness, albeit removed from your immediate attention. But they are there none the less. Suppose you were in a different situation, perhaps interviewing a subordinate at work, and certain outside concerns kept creeping into your consciousness, distracting you from full attention to your conversation.

The broth of the moment is mixed with ingredients of no immediate relevance. You are neither here nor there. You experience various confusing emotions and thoughts that dilute your concentration on the task at hand. Under such circumstances you cannot possibly do your best. Outside concerns compete with present interests. How do we overcome this, so we can advance through our moments with full attention, commitment and enjoyment? This may be our greatest challenge!

The working mother can be torn by conflict, making it difficult to do quality work and be a good mother at the same time. A continuing health problem can be a constant source of fear, confusion and distraction from our work. Meeting these challenges requires what we have called Focused Action. We must make choices that lead to Focused Action. When at work, pay attention to your work. When at home, pay attention to home life. When playing golf — well, have a good time.

Feeling connected is very much what living in the zone is about. Mental, physical, emotional aspects of your total being are fully related to your actions in each moment. You are doing what you want to do, and you are doing it well. Awareness of your inner voices, of your personal concerns, of your compelling interests and deepest desires, is essential to living in the zone. You are what you do. Do what you do best. Do it well.

Notes

NOTES

IN THE ZONE

[1] P. Ekman *Facial Expressions of Emotion: New Findings, New Questions, Psychological Science*, 1992, 3:34 - 38.

RELAXATION

[1] Dan Millman, *The Inner Athlete* (Walpole, NH: Stillpoint Publishers, 1979), pp. 69-70.

[2] In an earlier publication, I introduced a method for deep relaxation called Relaxation Therapy. Included in this method are instructions on how to use deep breathing in the Position of Comfort. Ray C. Mulry, *Tension Management & Relaxation* (St. Louis, MO: C.V. Mosby Company, 1982).

[3] The effects of stress on learning are documented by Carla Hannaford in *Smart Moves: Why Learning Is Not All In Your Head* (Arlington, VA: Great Ocean Publishers, 1995), pp. 160-165.

[4] Deepak Chopra, *Quantum Healing, Exploring The Frontiers of Mind/ Body Medicine* (New York: Bantam Books, 1990), pp. 66-67.

[5] Carla Hannaford, *Smart Moves: Why Learning Is Not All In Your Head* (Arlington, VA: Great Ocean Publishers, 1995), p. 170.

[6] Nikolai I. Tarasov, *Ballet Technique For The Male Dancer* (Garden City, NY: Doubleday, 1985), p. 39.

[7] Niel Glixon, *Ballet Without Tears* (New York: The Fowler School of Classical Ballet, 1968), p. 13.

[8] William L. Stephens, Jr., *Rifle Marksmanship* (New York: A.S. Barnes & Company, 1941), pp. 70-71.

[9] Sally Swift, *Centered Riding* (New York: St. Martin's/Marek, 1985), pp. 15-16.

[10] Albert J. Fracht and Emmett Robinson, *Sing Well, Speak Well* (Brooklyn, NY: Remsen Press, 1984), p. 6.

[11] Arthur L. Manchester *Twelve Lessons In The Fundamentals Of Voice Production* (New York: Ditson Company, 1977), pp. 12-13.

BALANCE

[1] Jacob, Ellen. *Dancing: A Guide for the Dancer You Can Be* (NY: Addison-Wesley, 1981), p. 227.

[2] *The Seven Samurai*, Directed by Akira Kurosawa (Toho Company, 1954).

[3] Y.K. Chen, *Tai-chi Ch'uan, Its Effects & Practical Applications* (North Hollywood, CA: Newcastle Publishing, 1979), p. 8.

[4] Jean-Claude Killy, *Skiing ... The Killy Way* (NY: Simon and Schuster, 1971), p. 126.

[5] Julius Palffy-Alpar, *Sword and Mask* (Philadelphia: F.A. Davis, 1967), p. viii.

FLEXIBILITY

[1] Quoted in Joe Hyams, *Zen In The Martial Arts* (NY: Bantam Books, 1979), p. 67.

[2] Swami Vishnudevananda, *The Complete Illustrated Book of Yoga* (NY: Bell Publishing Co., 1959), p. 199.

[3] Gia-fu Feng, *Tai Chi, A Way of Centering and I Ching* (NY: Collier Books, 1970), p. 93.

[4] Michael J. Alter, *Science of Stretching* (Champaign, IL: Human Kinetics Books, 1988), p.101.

[5] Cecil M. Colwin, *Swimming into the 21st Century* (Champaign, IL: Leisure Press, 1992), p. 211.

[6] James Gleick, *Genius: The Life and Science of Richard Feynman* (NY: Pantheon Books, 1992), p. 19.

[7] James D. Watson, *The Double Helix* (NY: New American Library, 1968), p. 112.

[8] Thomas S. Kuhn, *The Structure of Scientific Revolutions* (Chicago: University of Chicago Press, 1962).

[9] David Gelernter, *The Muse in the Machine, Computerizing the Poetry of Human Thought* (NY: The Free Press, 1994).

[10] Ronald W. Clark, *Einstein: The Life and Times* (NY: Avon Books, 1971), p. 118.

FOCUS

[1] Ray Mulry, *Power Breathing, Videocassette Training Program* (Incline Village, NV: American Network Services, Inc., 1987).

[2] Kenneth Kushner, *One Arrow, One Life* (New York and London: Arkana, 1988), pp. 102-103.

[3] Carla Hannaford, *Smart Moves: Why Learning Is Not All In Your Head* (Arlington, VA: Great Ocean Publishers, 1995), pp. 174-175.

LIVING IN THE ZONE

[1] Hathaway, M.L. & Hathaway, *Yoga For Athletics* (Chicago: Contemporary Books, 1978).

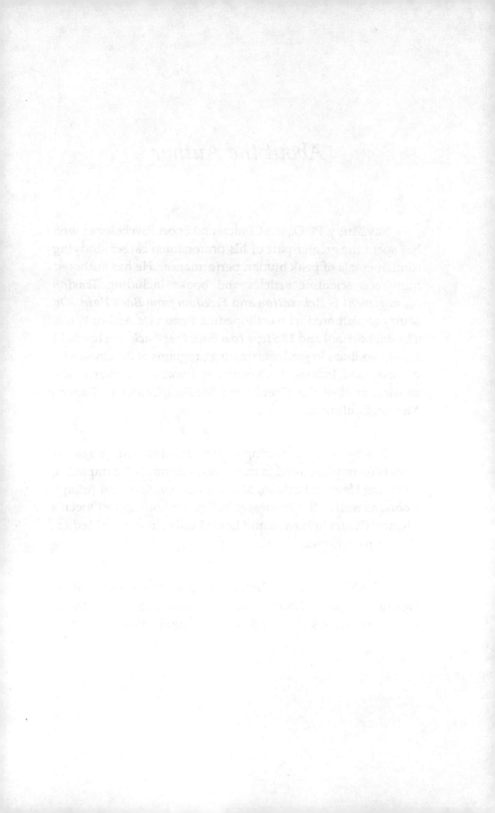

About the Author

Ray Mulry, Ph.D., is a Clinical and Sport Psychologist who has spent the greater part of his professional career studying fundamentals of peak human performance. He has authored numerous scientific articles and books including *Tension Management & Relaxation* and *Freedom from Back Pain*. Dr. Mulry co-authored with orthopedic surgeon Dr. Arthur White *The Back School* and *12 Steps to a Pain Free Back*. He has held faculty positions in graduate training programs of the University of Texas and Indiana University, and was a member of the medical staff of the Eisenhower Medical Center in Rancho Mirage, California.

Ray Mulry's pioneering human development programs have been implemented in numerous Fortune 500 companies, including Hewlett-Packard, Marriott Corporation, and Adolph Coors, as well as the Tennessee Valley Authority, The Queen's Medical Center in Hawaii and Loma Linda University Medical Center in California.

Dr. Mulry makes his home in Incline Village, Lake Tahoe, Nevada, where he directs American Network Services, Inc., a management consulting and training organization.